The Dynamic Assessment of Language Learning

This is a practical, accessible manual for Speech and Language Therapists, Educational Psychologists and Educators who assess children with language impairments, explaining how and why to implement Dynamic Assessment and giving you a huge range of ready-to-use, practical tools. Where standardised assessments simply identify deficits, Dynamic Assessment also identifies the child's potential to learn by allowing for prompts from you, during the assessment, thus better informing your decisions about appropriate interventions and strategies to help the children you work with.

What does this manual offer?

- Provides a concise introduction to the principles of Dynamic Assessment to make clear the enormous benefits of applying this approach to the assessment of language.

- Presents a full example of a Dynamic Assessment of Sentence Structure (DASS) to demonstrate how the principles are implemented and the findings applied to plan more effective interventions. All the materials for the DASS are included so that you can use this assessment immediately.

- Includes numerous templates, generic prompt sheets, score sheets and materials that you can adapt for use in Dynamic Assessments that you devise yourself.

Written by Dr Natalie Hasson, a highly experienced Speech and Language Therapist who leads the field in researching the Dynamic Assessment of language, this is the only Dynamic Assessment manual of its kind.

Dr Natalie Hasson has many years' international experience as a clinical Speech and Language Therapist and as a Clinical Tutor for language development and language disorder modules at City University London. Her particular research interest is the Dynamic Assessment of language disorders in children, and she has published a wide range of research papers in this area.

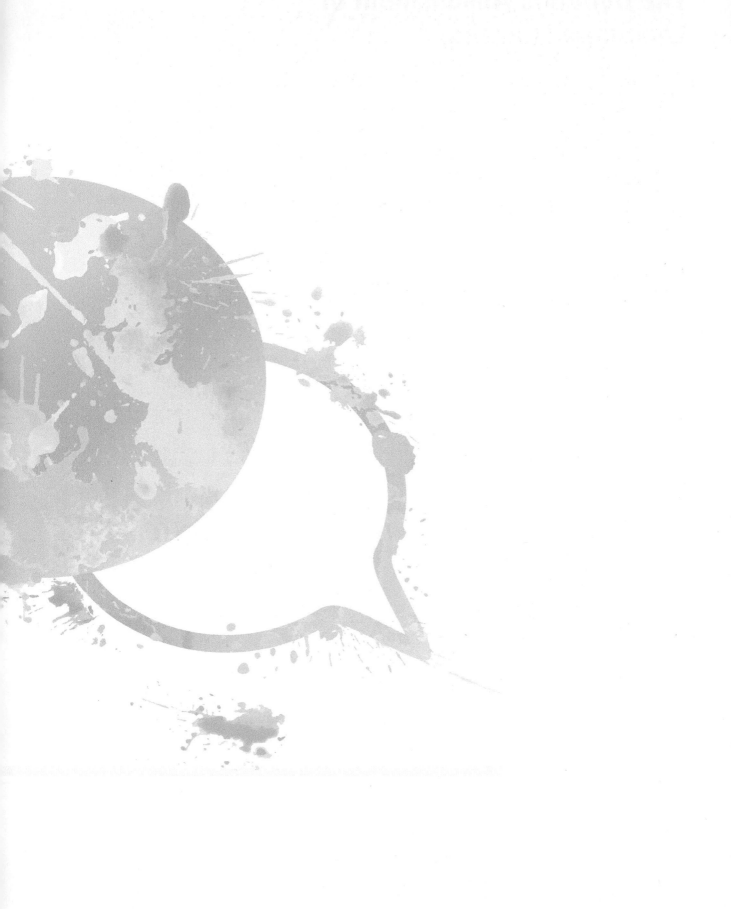

THE DYNAMIC ASSESSMENT OF LANGUAGE LEARNING

NATALIE HASSON

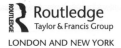

Routledge
Taylor & Francis Group

LONDON AND NEW YORK

First published 2018
by Routledge
2 Park Square, Milton Park, Abingdon, Oxon OX14 4RN

and by Routledge
711 Third Avenue, New York, NY 10017

Routledge is an imprint of the Taylor & Francis Group, an informa business

British Library Cataloguing-in-Publication Data
A catalogue record for this book is available from the British Library

Library of Congress Cataloging-in-Publication Data
A catalog record for this book has been requested

ISBN: 978-1-911186-18-2 (pbk)
ISBN: 978-1-315-17542-3 (ebk)

Typeset in Univers
by Apex CoVantage, LLC

For Nathan who has made it all possible.

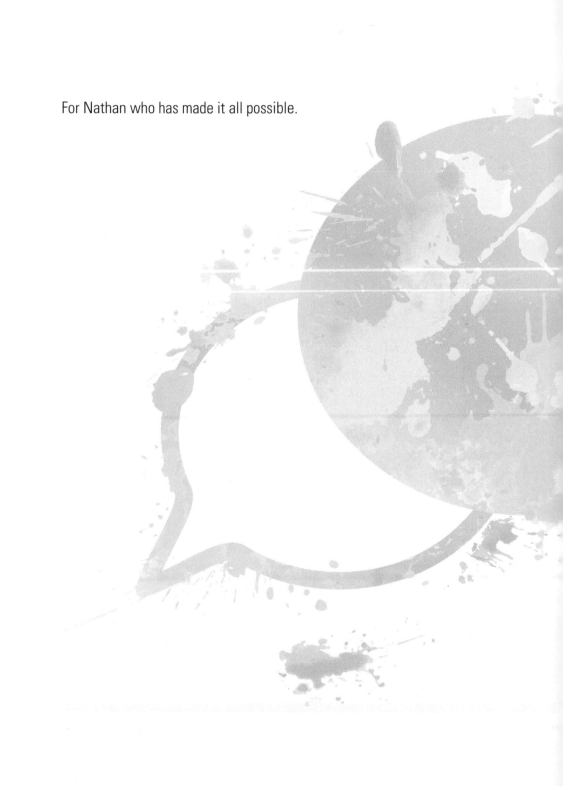

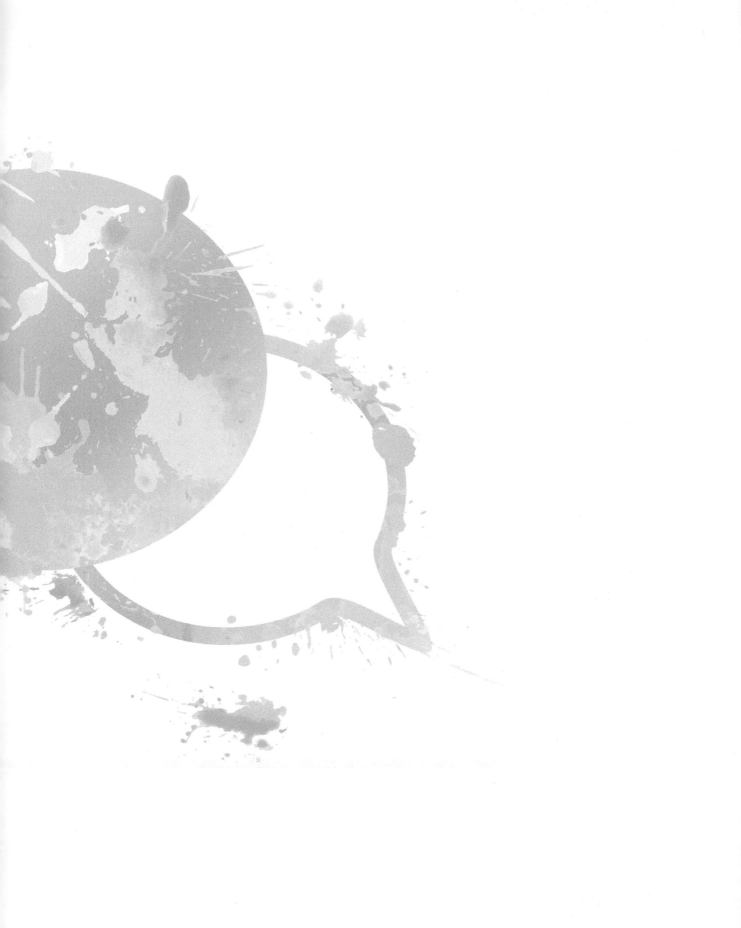

Contents

Acknowledgements

My sincere thanks go to many people who have contributed directly or indirectly to the development of this work:

Ruth Deutsch

Elizabeth Peña

Nicola Botting

Barbara Dodd

Bernard Camilleri

Stephen Parsons

I would also like to thank the numerous speech and language therapists and the children whose contributions to my research made this work possible.

Finally, I thank my family and particularly my husband, Nathan, who encouraged me every step of the way.

Chapter 1
Introduction

The dynamic assessment of language learning

About this resource

What does it contain?

Who is it for?

Who can be assessed?

Children with language disorders

Planning intervention

The dynamic assessment of language learning

Dynamic assessment (DA), as we will see, is an umbrella term for a range of assessment models and methods. What they all have in common is the intention to do a small amount of teaching *within* the assessment and to gauge how an individual responds to that intervention. This then enables the assessor to see how well the individual is *able to learn*, rather than how much he has already learnt.

The approach has been adapted from the assessment of cognition or intelligence, where it is an alternative (or addendum) to IQ testing. The DA of language works really well, because the process of learning language is readily differentiated from the language that has been learnt.

So, for example, instead of a test asking whether a child uses past-tense endings incorrectly, we might ask the following:

- Does the child understand the task he is being required to do? What does the child think it is?

- Does the child understand the language being directed to him?

- Is the child familiar with the pictures or materials being used?
- Does the child have a concept of time or events being in the past?
- Does the child know the usual past-tense ending?
- Does the child know when to apply it? Does he know the rules?
- Can the child produce it?

And also

- Does the child know when he has got it right?
- Does the child think it is hard? Which parts does he perceive as difficult?

And, most importantly,

- What kind of intervention does the child need in order to use the past tense correctly?
- How readily did the child grasp the teaching? Did he need a lot of repetition? What else can I do to help him achieve it?
- Can the child easily generalise what he has learnt? How much help does he need to do that?

We find out about these things by giving structured prompts or cues and by asking specific questions. We also *mediate* to enable the child to find and understand the concepts himself, appreciate their relevance and when they can be applied to other examples. In this volume, we will learn more about how to mediate effectively to achieve these things.

At the end of the process, the DA can give information about how the child learns, what strategies he finds useful and how he understands the process of learning language structures. The principles of devising a DA can be applied to the assessment of a wide range of language structures in both first and second language learners in much the same way as a battery of standardised language tests is frequently used. The findings will be very useful and practical, leading the assessor or therapist towards devising effective individual language intervention programmes.

About this resource

What does it contain?

The content of this volume is intended to give you, the practitioner, the background to DA so that you can understand the principles and devise your own assessments. This is because there are very few published dynamic tests of language. DAs don't use norms and therefore don't need to be standardised on large populations. The scoring is standardised enough for you to be able to compare one child with another, if you want to use the tests for this purpose, or, for example, you need to prioritise children for intervention. The main application, however, is clinical, so you can adapt your intervention for each child, maximise their learning in sessions and hypothesise about the amount of intervention they might need.

Chapter 2 introduces the field of DA and gives a broad overview of methods that are included. The rationale and evidence base for DA are briefly reviewed.

Chapter 3 will address the specific aspects of language that may be assessed and how to analyse the tasks and grade the prompts. It will also cover how to devise test-teach-retest procedures with mediated interventions. The scoring of procedures will be covered in Chapter 4.

All of this instruction will be illustrated in Chapter 5 by a description of one of the available language tests, the Dynamic Assessment of Sentence Structure (DASS) (Hasson, Dodd and Botting 2012).

Chapter 6 explores the application of the findings of the DA to the planning of intervention, again with illustrations from the DASS. All of the DASS materials and templates can be found in Appendix A, so you can use that instrument as it stands. Alternatively, you can use the information, scales and templates in Appendix B to construct your own test procedures, or the references in Appendix C to follow up other applications of DA to adults and other clinical populations.

Who is it for?

This guide is for any professional engaged in the assessment of language. It is not limited to speech and language therapists (SLTs), but may also be used by educational psychologists (EPs), or indeed clinical or cognitive psychologists and educationalists including teachers, special needs teachers or special education needs and disabilities co-ordinators (SENDCos). The only limitation is that the assessor needs a good grasp of language structure and a clear idea of the component skills in a language task.

Who can be assessed?

DA can be used on a wide range of typical and clinical populations. It may be used with adults with a range of cognitive and linguistic difficulties (see references in Appendix C). Most of the examples throughout the text will be about children. For convenience, individual child clients to be assessed are referred to as 'he' in this text, and the assessor is referred to throughout as 'she'.

Because the tests are not normed on a specific population, they can be used on the clinical groups for whom standardised tests do not apply, for example, those with hearing losses;

autism spectrum disorders;

learning difficulties;

attention deficits;

emotional and behavioural difficulties; and

bilingual or multilingual children.

Many of the prompts and questions will require the children to have a certain level of language. However, since the instructions are not necessarily scripted and any words may be used, the assessor can simplify the language as much as is needed for a particular child, or use signs, symbols or pictures to support language. Along with selecting the appropriate language targets for the test, the cues and prompts can be made age appropriate.

Children as young as three can be assessed, but of course the questions about metalinguistics, such as "Which word would you use . . .?" or "What sound is on the end?" would be limited. Similarly, you wouldn't be able to ask metacognitive questions such as "How did you do that?" or "How did you know?"

Some work has been done on DA with children who use sign language, and these are also referenced in Appendix C.

Children with language disorders

Children with language difficulties present in many different ways. No single explanation for the difficulties has yet been found that accounts for all the different presentations of language difficulties. There are, for example, so many children with difficulties in grammar, tenses, word order and word endings that linguistic theories have been proposed to explain the poor processing of grammatical features and rules. However, these do not adequately account for the deficits in phonological working memory and non-word repetition. A more cognitive or processing based explanation is required. These theories imply that some more general processing skills such as speed of processing and working memory may also be involved.

Recent debate about the labelling of language impairments has highlighted problems with definition. The assumption that language impairments can be identified while non-verbal abilities are normal is no longer considered valid. The relationship between verbal and non-verbal skills is complex and changes over time.

One possible label for the language difficulties encountered by children is 'language learning impairment'. This term implies a problem or difficulty with the *learning* of the language system. This definition of the condition is consistent with an approach to assessment that looks at the process of learning. DAs aim to do exactly that: consider what the child understands the task to be and how he approaches it. They look at what strategies a child uses to decode language and what cues help him to learn words and structures. Is a lot of repetition useful? Or visual associations? Signs? Rules?

The preferred label is 'developmental language disorder' (DLD). This places emphasis on the developmental aspect, that is, that the child has not learnt language in the typical way or at the usual speed. We will see that some of the theory underpinning DA refers to inadequate *mediation* in the early years. This means that some children have not had sufficient quality input and guidance to enable them to master the language. Some children require more input and mediation, and DA seeks to identify the facilitation that is needed to support the development of language in an individual child.

Because the format of a DA is flexible and there are different formats to choose, you can devise an assessment to probe different language structures and the skills that are necessary for those structures to be learnt correctly. More detailed examples of procedures will be given in Chapter 3 and Appendix B.

Planning intervention

Standardised language tests are very good at telling us what language a child does not use correctly. For example, we may see that he fails to use the correct pronouns 'he' or 'she'. Or he leaves out the auxiliary verb 'is' and produces sentences such as '*he running*' and '*mummy sleeping now*'. Although the tests do not claim to make recommendations for intervention, the nature of the findings leads therapists to address the errors. So they target pronouns and teach the child to use 'he' when they see a picture of a boy doing an action and 'she' for a girl. They practice sentences that start with 'she' and not 'her'. These programmes, which Law *et al.* (2008) termed 'skills based', are primarily used with younger children and achieve the intended results; the child eventually produces correct sentences, and the therapist moves on to the next target.

What these therapies do not necessarily do is teach the child to understand the principles of the application of the rules. Older children are more often treated in this way, using what Law *et al.* (2008) identified as 'metalinguistic approaches'. The best-known, evidence-based metalinguistic therapies are Colourful Semantics (Bryan 1997) and Shape Coding (Ebbels 2007). These make it much more explicit to the child what functions the words in the sentence perform and how they are to be arranged. A grasp of the principles enables an individual to formulate and apply rules and generalise what they have learnt. This is the process of learning.

DAs find out much more detailed information about a child's capabilities than a static test. Asking probing questions and giving clues enables the assessor to find out whether the child understands the task, the underlying concepts involved, the rules and whether he is able to generalise the knowledge to new examples. It can also be used to find out whether the child recognises when the structure is used correctly or when it is wrong. Finally, it also looks at the response of the child to the intervention. Are they willing to listen and learn? Do they catch on quickly, or do they require lots of repetition? Do they need visual support to enable them to remember? This detailed information helps the therapist or teacher plan a more effective intervention programme. We will take a closer look at this in Chapter 6.

References

Bryan, A. (1997) 'Colourful semantics', Chiat, S., Law, J. and Marshall, J. (eds) *Language disorders in children and adults: Psycholinguistic approaches to therapy*, Whurr, London.

Ebbels, S. (2007) 'Teaching grammar to school-aged children with specific language impairment using shape coding', *Child Language Teaching and Therapy*, 23(1), pp. 67–93.

Hasson, N., Dodd, B. and Botting, N. (2012) 'Dynamic Assessment of Sentence Structure (DASS): Design and evaluation of a novel procedure for assessment of syntax in children with language impairments', *International Journal of Language and Communication Disorders*, 47(3), pp. 285–299.

Law, J., Campbell, C., Roulstone, S., Adams, C. and Boyle, J. (2008) 'Mapping practice onto theory: The speech and language practitioner's construction of receptive language impairment', *International Journal of Language & Communication Disorders*, 43(3), pp. 245–263.

Chapter 2
Theory and rationale

What is dynamic assessment?

The term 'dynamic assessment' is used interchangeably with other terms such as 'interactive assessment' and 'learning potential assessment'. The most defining aspect, however, is "*active intervention by the examiners and assessment of examinees' response to intervention*" (Haywood and Lidz 2007 p. 1). This is a really broad definition; it encompasses all types of interventions within an assessment and any occasion on which the tester "*does more than give instructions, pose questions and record responses*" (Haywood and Lidz 2007 p. 1).

DAs are usually contrasted to 'static' 'standardised' or 'normative' assessments. This implies that DA procedures are none of these things, but this is not strictly true. European researchers have devised dynamic tests that are standardised and psychometrically validated (Hessels, Berger and Bosson 2008). The more useful contrast to a DA is a *static* test that looks at an individual's independent performance on a given task at a given point in time. This is the model of language tests with which therapists are most familiar.

The focus of a DA is not entirely on the *content* of the test, that is, the items of language that the individual knows, rather it looks at *process* or how the individual learns. What kinds of stimuli are useful to him? Verbal explanation? Visual pictures? Following an example? Does he recognise that a rule is required and know what that rule is? Does he have the confidence to try? Does he just guess randomly and use trial and error, or is there systematic hypothetical thinking? How much help does he need?

It is not recommended that static tests are replaced by DA. Rather, the two procedures are seen to be complementary and useful in combination. This way you can both identify or classify an individual with a disorder, as compared to his peers, and determine his potential to learn from instruction.

The theory

The first basis for DA came from Vygotsky. Vygotsky (1986) stressed the role of others in the environment, who present, instruct and mediate meanings to the developing child. These external instructions have to be actively internalised and assimilated by the child, who cannot remain a passive recipient of information, but rather has to be involved in making the meanings his own.

Vygotsky described the development of a child's thinking as an ever-changing system of mental functions. The sources of this change and development are experiential learning, formal learning and mediation through other human beings. The more basic concepts are learnt by experience, and these are gradually refined and advanced by formal teaching and through the mediation of others, usually parents, carers, siblings, peers or teachers.

The zone of proximal development (ZPD) is one of Vygotsky's best-known constructs. It links to the role of others facilitating a child's learning and aims to measure how much more a child can achieve with support from someone else, compared to what he can manage independently. It is similar to the more familiar concept of 'stimulability', that is, "Is it possible to facilitate an improved performance through teaching, and how much teaching effort does it take?"

Some children will grasp what is being taught easily and manage it on their own, while others will not be able to succeed even with facilitation; in other words, the skill is not within their ZPD.

DA is focused on this measurement of the ZPD. It doesn't measure what the child can already do, but looks at the level he can reach with assistance and the nature of the assistance that is required.

At this point enter Feuerstein.

Reuven Feuerstein believed that all individuals have the capacity to change – a theory he termed 'structural cognitive modifiability' (Feuerstein *et al.* 2003). The aim of his clinical work was to determine how to effect that change, in other words, what kind of input was needed for an individual to achieve new skills. He believed that it is the quality of the interaction with others, as well as the nature of the stimuli, that is responsible for facilitating significant change. So it is not enough to present a developing child with stimuli, even carefully chosen ones, unless there is high-quality input to shape their learning.

Feuerstein called this high-quality input the 'mediated learning experience' or MLE. He and his followers have described in detail what qualities an interaction must have in order to be described as truly mediational, which we will look at in detail in the next section.

So the common theme is the input of others into the learning process. DAs look at this learning process. How we actually measure the learning varies, but there is always a role for input within the assessment process. In many ways this makes sense, the interaction between client and therapist is always important in therapy and a crucial aim for intervention, yet we are inclined to assess in the most artificial and contrived way, giving no feedback or cues to the person being tested. We know that this doesn't enable their best performance, yet this is what we use. It is not really surprising that standardised language tests have low reliability (Dockrell 2001).

How does it work?

There are a number of different ways in which DA works. Which one you adopt depends primarily on your client and on what you would like to get out of the assessment. So if you assess a child and have to decide whether he is a priority for immediate intervention, you need to be able to compare different children to each other, and you need a fairly standard procedure and reliable, preferably quantified, scoring. If you are doing research, these criteria are even more important. Counting the number of prompts given is usually the way forward, and careful grading of the prompts is important. If your main aim is to discover how an individual child processes language and how best to facilitate his improvement, you could go with a more individualised, mediated programme that reveals qualitative guidelines for therapy. Or you might rate the intensity of intervention given, or the responsiveness of the child to your intervention, using a rating scale. However, you can also 'mix and match' these methods, or even combine them for any particular case.

A closer look at the methods

Test-train-retest

Early assessments in the DA tradition seem to have been addressed to equal opportunities. They aimed to give applicants from all backgrounds an equal chance in their applications for study and employment (Budoff 1987). Individuals were tested, and then trained in the basic skills they would need and may not have had the opportunity to experience before, and then retested. High scores on the retest were considered more fair evaluations of ability than the pre-test, which reflected both ability and experience. The procedures also gave rise to *gain* scores: the difference between pre-test and post-test scores, which reflected the individual's ability to learn or benefit from training. In this way, *potential to learn* was identified.

This is essentially also what therapists do in stimulability tests, or trial therapy: identify the difficulty in a static test, try out some therapy and see whether the individual improves. Test-train-retest remains a fundamental procedure in DA. It is not very new or very different from other systems, but because a trial procedure is standardised and condensed into the assessment, it is less time consuming and more useful.

Graduated prompts

Building on the idea of Vygotsky's ZPD, we can see that children who display readiness to learn a task benefit from intervention in that task, while those with less readiness have a 'narrower' ZPD and require more specific direction to achieve success in the task. Campione and Brown (1987) measured the ZPD by measuring the amount of help a child needed to complete a task. They gave a child a task or problem to solve. If the child failed, they gave the child a clue and continued to add clues as needed, for as long as the child struggled. The clues started broadly, and became more and more specific and directed towards the problem. When the task was complete, they counted the number of cues given. They then gave another item and repeated the procedure to see whether the child had learnt from the previous example and fewer cues would be needed.

The notion of giving the *least* supportive cues first is different from traditional approaches to language teaching in which the target is first modelled for the client. The process is more of trying to get the individual to problem solve for himself, with as little help as possible. You would gradually build up to the most directive cue, which is a model for the child to imitate. If a child needs this level of prompting, we know that he will require more intensive intervention in order to learn a target.

The requirement for the assessor is to analyse the task in detail and construct a hierarchy of cues from least to most helpful. It takes a bit of restructuring to save the complete model until last.

Mediational intervention

The approach of Feuerstein is more clinical in emphasis. He devised a battery of tests of cognitive function, the Learning Propensity Assessment Device (LPAD), a few of which have verbal stimuli and may be useful assessments of language (for example, the '16-word memory test' (Feuerstein *et al.* 1979)). Most of the instruments use a test-teach-retest format in which the teach phase comprises different types of facilitations, including mediational intervention. This is a specific type of intervention that we will look at in the next section.

The different tests in the battery vary considerably in structure, and Feuerstein's procedures allow for mediation at different phases in the test procedure. There is, for example, preparatory or pre-test mediation that enables the assessor to orientate the learner to the task and materials, as well as teaching any prerequisite content. Mediation *during* the test consists of regulating behaviour, inputting knowledge, providing feedback and facilitating appropriate responses, or there is mediation *after* the performance, regulating behaviour, giving feedback and encouraging reflective insights. Some tests consist of several trials that enable the individual to learn successively from repetition and practice, with or without explicit feedback (e.g. the 16-word memory test), while others provide additional learning opportunities. In this way, the battery allows for probing of responsiveness to different models of learning and cueing, enabling the assessor to gain a composite profile of the learner's abilities.

There is consistency between the graduated prompts method and the mediational input of Feuerstein in the way in which the programme is constructed, that is, from the broadest, least directive cues to the more specific and directive. Feuerstein *et al.* (2002) called this a scale of 'Required Mediational Intervention' (RMI). In his descriptions of RMI (see Appendix B01), it can be seen that when the adult prompt is least directive (level 9), the child is more active as a problem solver, and as the assessor intervenes more (level 0), the child is seen as more passive.

There are valuable principles embedded in Feuerstein's test procedures that lead towards the detailed and individualised knowledge of a person's needs for support. Some of these will be familiar and already in the repertoire of language therapists, while incorporating others into the test procedure will require some practice and reflection.

Feedback

This approach was devised by Carlson and Wiedl (1992) and termed 'Testing the Limits'. Essentially, the assessors experimented with giving different amounts of feedback to the individual doing a task. Generally, in standardised tests, no feedback at all is given, but Carlson and Wiedl found that if detailed feedback was given during an assessment task, performance on successive items improved. In fact, when very detailed feedback that included the child explaining why he responded in the way he did, and verbalising alternative strategies was used, improvements were greater.

The measurement in such a procedure is based on the improvement from one item to another. If a child is seen to use what he has learnt to transfer to the next item without any prompting from the assessor, he is clearly a good learner.

Elizabeth Peña, whose research we will meet in the next section, adapted the idea of feedback into what she termed a 'clinical interview' (Gutierrez-Clellen and Peña 2001). In this procedure, which was used with bilingual children, after the test items were answered, the assessor formulated questions to help the children explain their answers and reflect on their knowledge.

The approach is very variable and cannot be scored, but it has good face validity and elicits a great deal of very useful qualitative information that can be used in planning interventions.

The interested reader can read up more on these and other methods from the reference list. The paper by Gutierrez-Clellen and Peña (2001) is an excellent starting point. Remember that a combination of methods can be used according to your needs.

What is mediated intervention?

Feuerstein identified the MLE as a specific kind of intervention that brings about permanent and pervasive cognitive changes in another individual (Feuerstein *et al.* 2003). In other words, it teaches them to think and process in a way that underpins their functioning from that time on. In the development of this theory, Feuerstein parallels the socio-cultural framework associated with Vygotsky in which the parents or caregivers of a child assume a central role. Although all children have access to some input, the quantity and quality of MLE varies, and according to Haywood (1993), inadequate MLE leads to inadequate cognitive development. The aim of remediational interventions is to supply MLE to redress the previous inadequacies.

In a mediated learning situation, the mediator shapes the experience of the learner by placing himself between the stimulus, or the experience, and the individual. He is thus able to help the learner attend selectively to relevant stimuli, focus on important aspects, process appropriately using comparisons and links to past experiences, and generalise the experience to new situations (Haywood 1993).

MLE is defined by the presence of a number of mediating behaviours. The most essential of these have been adapted from Feuerstein by Carol Lidz (1991, 2003) as follows:

Mediation of intentionality – conveying to the child that you intend to help him improve. This is important but also unusual in SLT for children in that the process is made very explicit to the learner. He cannot passively submit to learning, but has to actively engage and play a part (termed '*reciprocity*') in the learning. He needs to know why he is there.

Mediation of meaning – the learner also needs to come to appreciate the importance of what he is learning. If he is aware of what he is learning and how it will benefit him, he engages more with the process. The assessor needs to communicate to the child the purpose of the lesson, which also maintains the child's involvement.

Mediation of transcendence – refers to linking the activity to other contexts in which the skill can be used, establishing 'cognitive bridges' between the task or activity and other related situations in which the same skill may be used. Reference may be made to past situations, or hypothetical future occasions when it may be useful.

Mediation of a feeling of competence – targeting praise so that the child learns what he has done well, learns that the tester has confidence in him and gains confidence in his own ability.

It can be seen that mediational intervention is very explicit. There is no sense of therapy being something that is done to the child; rather, he must actively engage in it. Part of the process is also therefore reflective and metacognitive; the child is asked to think about what he is doing and how he is managing.

According to Haywood (1993 p. 31), mediators have the following functions:

1   *Supply the information that may be needed to learn relationships or find solutions.*

2   *Ask questions – to elicit rather than give answers.*

3   *Guide learning by arranging and directing sequences of experiences in a developmental fashion or in increasing difficulty.*

4   *Bring about induction of rules by calling attention to similarities among events or examples.*

5   *Facilitate application of rules.*

6   *Build confidence of children.*

7   *Maintain a metacognitive emphasis – focus attention on the child's own thinking processes and encourage him to do the same.*

Therapists are often wary of asking too many questions, especially as they may put a child under pressure to perform. Mediational intervention includes a great deal of questioning, but because it is carefully graded and scaffolded, there is less pressure, and there is more of a sense of joint problem solving than a test that one must pass. Many of the questions, such as reflective ones, have no correct answer e.g. *"How did you know that?"*

How do I mediate? (Haywood 1993)

Ask process questions (usually containing 'how')
How did you know?
How else could you do that?
How can you find out?

Bridge to different applications
Elicit ideas from the children rather than telling them
e.g. When is another time you could do that?

Challenge the child to justify his answers, both right and wrong responses
Why did you do it like that?
That's right, but how else could you do it?
Why is that way better than this?

Teach about rules
If we have that and that, what rule can we make? Does it apply to this?
Would it help to have a rule here?
Would a rule help us to know what to do?

Emphasise order, system, sequence and strategy
Try to facilitate a predictable approach and enable planning
Use a timetable for the day and/or the session.
Reduce trial-and-error behaviour, guessing and random answers.

Create task-intrinsic motivation (Feuerstein)
Help the child to appreciate that the task is meaningful and motivate him to complete a task by emphasizing the achievement

Grading the prompts given to a child yields a great deal of information about how best to help him to achieve targets in therapy. However, mediational intervention yields even more information about how a child thinks, processes and approaches problem solving in a task. Omitting the challenge questions, the reflective questions and those about transfer to other contexts leads to missed opportunities to really understand the child and how to help him learn.

We will cover more practical examples of mediation in the next chapter.

What evidence is there for DA of language?

Studies using a range of dynamic methods have addressed the learning of different aspects of the language system. Many studies by educationalists have attempted to predict educational progress and reading skills using DAs of phonological processing and word learning in order to plan programmes. Studies by speech and language therapists have aimed to differentiate children with language disorders from those with English as an additional language (EAL or bilingual children) through DAs of vocabulary, word learning, expressive language and narrative.

A selection of studies is presented here and interested readers are encouraged to follow up on studies from the reference list.

Phonology

Dynamic screening of phonological awareness (DSPA), Bridges and Catts (2011)

A dynamic version of the Static Deletion Test (SDT), which requires the child to delete a syllable from a given word (e.g. 'say cowboy without cow') or delete the initial consonant (C) from CVC and CCVC words (e.g. 'say bread without the 'b') found that

- DA added to prediction of reading available from static test; and
- DSPA significant predictor of word reading outcomes, SDT, was not significant.

Non-verbal phoneme deletion test. Gillam et al. (2011)

Assessed phonological awareness (PA) skill in children with complex communication disorders unable to give a verbal response. The study found

- results correlated with static form of test and with measures of word-level reading;
- non-verbal test of phoneme deletion was valid and useful for non-verbal and unintelligible children; and
- DA aspect reveals important diagnostic information about PA skill as well as prescriptive information about the kinds of errors a child is making and what concepts need to be addressed in intervention.

Morphology

Morphological analysis in school-age children. Larsen and Nippold (2007)
and
Morphological analysis in context versus isolation. Ram et al. (2013)

Used the graduated prompt method to determine if children can derive meanings of morphologically complex words. The study found

- developmental trend – older children required fewer prompts;
- children in grade 3 (mean age 9.1) were able to identify and name parts of words correctly;
- children in grade 3 are able to determine meanings of complex words from parts with adult scaffolding; they are able to benefit from support and are modifiable;
- children were able to use cues from sentence context to determine meanings (less need for adult support); and
- DA is useful in determining strategies used by children.

Vocabulary

DA of receptive vocabulary. Camilleri and Law (2007)

Developed in order to compare the performance of monolingual English speakers with children with EAL and of typically developing children (TD) with those referred to SLT services. The study found

- ability to differentiate between TD children and those referred to SLT services;
- equal performance between monolingual children and children with EAL, whose static scores on the British Picture Vocabulary Scales (BPVS) differed; and
- suggests that the static test may not be suitable for children with EAL and risks overdiagnosing them as language impaired.

DA of word learning skills to identify language impairment in bilingual children. Kapantzoglou, Restrepo, and Thompson (2012)

The study found

- findings consistent with other studies – ratings of modifiability improve classification accuracy;
- children with primary language impairment have limited abilities to fast map new words – increased exposures reduce the difference; and
- DA useful in differential diagnosis in bilingual children – potential to learn words indicative of overall language ability.

Word learning from reading. Steele and Watkins (2010)

Children with learning language difficulty and typical language development (TLD) both expected to show improved word learning with more exposures to target words and with more context clues. The study found

- the need for DA justified by higher scores with contextual clues – children were more proficient than was observable through their independent efforts;
- contextual clues were helpful to all children, although TLD children received more of a benefit; and
- children may be taught to use context to determine meaning and may be taught skills of definition.

Two-word level

DA of two-word level. Olswang, Bain and Johnson (1992)

Two children, aged 32 and 35 months, using single words only were assessed via a hierarchy of prompts and transfer tasks to determine the potential to progress to combining two words in various semantic relationships. The study found

- different potential for change confirmed by subsequently different rates of gain during the trial intervention period.

DA as a predictor of language change. Olswang and Bain (1996)

Twenty-one children from 31 to 36 months at the single-word stage and identified as having expressive language impairments. Language was measured in terms of mean length of utterance and proportional change over the intervention period calculated. The study found that

- individual static tests were not good predictors of language change; and
- DA scores had the highest correlations with proportional change index and accurately predicted children whose language would or would not change significantly during the treatment study.

Narrative

Classification ability of a DA of narrative. Peña (et al. 2006)

Examined the classification ability of a DA of narrative ability in first and second grade school children.

Two parallel wordless storybooks were used as pre- and post-tests.

Two sessions of individualised mediational intervention were carried out in the 'teach' phase.

Ratings of modifiability were carried out after the second intervention session.

The study found that

- all children performed better on the post-test after the two sessions of MLE, but the TD children showed greater gains than those with language impairment (LI);

- pre-test measures of narrative did not accurately classify TD and LI children; and
- the best single predictor was the clinician's modifiability rating, which was seen as consistent with the aims of DA, which are to assess responsiveness to instruction.

Assessment of Bilingual children

DA to assess children from different cultural groups.
Peña and Iglesias (1992)

Used a DA, including MLE, to assess children from culturally different (CLD) groups
The study found that

- post-test scores and modifiability ratings were useful to differentiate between typically developing children and those with language disorder.

DA to determine language impairments in CLD children. Peña (2000)

Clinician modifiability ratings were a useful, nonbiased means of determining diagnosis of LI in CLD children.

Reducing test bias through dynamic assessment of children's word learning ability. Peña, Iglesias and Lidz (2001)

Preschool CLD children were assessed in word learning.
The pre-test-teach-post-test method, with mediated strategies for naming in the teach phase was used. The study found that

- post-test scores and modifiability ratings differentiated the typically developing children from those with low language ability; and
- DA methods were more predictive in this differentiation than static pre-test scores, which have been shown to overdiagnose children with CLD as language impaired.

Discriminating disorder from difference using dynamic assessment with bilingual children. Hasson, Camilleri, Jones, Smith, and Dodd (2013)

Dynamic Assessment of Preschoolers' Proficiency in Learning English (DAPPLE) consists of vocabulary learning, sentence structure learning and phonology, all with brief test-teach-retest procedures. Trialled on 12 children referred by SLT and 14 with no known history, all bilingual and aged four to five. The study found the following:

- vocab – referred children needed more prompting to identify words and retained fewer words on post-test;

- expressive grammar – referred children needed more prompts and produced shorter clauses on post-test; and

- phonology – referred children produced fewer words accurately on pre- and post-test and were less consistent in trials.

The study concluded that DAPPLE data differentiated two groups, and it is a useful addition to tests of bilingual children.

In summary, there is research evidence in support of DA as a method for finding out more about the skills used by children with language impairments and how they differ from typically developing children, determining the presence of language impairments in bilingual children and as a predictor of learning ability in very young children. Ongoing research is establishing DA as an evidence-based approach to assessment, diagnosis, differential diagnosis and intervention planning.

References

Bridges, M.S., and Catts, H.W. (2011) 'The use of a dynamic screening of phonological awareness to predict risk for reading disabilities in kindergarten children', *Journal of Learning Disabilities*, 44(4), pp. 330–338.

Budoff, M. (1987) 'The validity of learning potential assessment', Lidz, C.S. (ed) *Dynamic assessment: An interactional approach to evaluating learning potential*, Guilford Press, New York.

Camilleri, B., and Law, J. (2007) 'Assessing children referred to speech and language therapy: Static and dynamic assessment of receptive vocabulary', *International Journal of Speech-Language Pathology*, 9(4), pp. 312–322.

Campione, J.C., and Brown, A.L. (1987) 'Linking dynamic assessment with school achievement', Lidz, C.S. (ed) *Dynamic assessment: An interactional approach to evaluating learning potential*, Guilford Press, New York.

Carlson, J.S., and Wiedl, K.H. (1992) 'Principles of dynamic assessment: The application of a specific model', *Learning and Individual Differences*, 4, pp. 153–166.

Dockrell, J.E. (2001) 'Assessing language skills in preschool children', *Child Psychology and Psychiatry Review*, 6(2), pp. 74–84.

Feuerstein, R., Feuerstein, R.S., Falik, L.H. and Rand, Y. (2002) *The dynamic assessment of cognitive modifiability: The learning propensity assessment device: Theory, instruments and techniques*, ICELP Press, Jerusalem.

Feuerstein, R., Haywood, H.C., Jensen, M.R., Rand, Y. and Hoffman, M.B. (1979) *LPAD tests – complex figure drawing – 16 word memory test*, Hadassah-WIZO-Canada Research Institute, Jerusalem.

Feuerstein, R., Rand, Y., Haywood, H.C., Kyram, L. and Hoffman, M.B. (2003) *Learning propensity assessment device manual*, ICELP Press, Jerusalem.

Gillam, S.L., Fargo, J., Foley, B. and Olszewski, A. (2011) 'A nonverbal phoneme deletion task administered in a dynamic assessment format', *Journal of Communication Disorders*, 44, pp. 236–245.

Gutierrez-Clellen, V.F., and Peña, E. (2001) 'Dynamic assessment of diverse children: A tutorial', *Language, Speech, and Hearing Services in Schools*, 32(4), pp. 212–224.

Hasson, N., Camilleri, B., Jones, C., Smith, J. and Dodd, B. (2013) 'Discriminating disorder from difference using dynamic assessment with bilingual children', *Child Language Teaching and Therapy*, 29(1), pp. 57–75.

Haywood, H.C. (1993) 'A mediational teaching style', *International Journal of Cognitive Education and Mediated Learning*, 3(1), pp. 27–38.

Haywood, H.C., and Lidz, C.S. (2007) *Dynamic assessment in practice: Clinical and educational applications*, Cambridge University Press, New York.

Hessels, M.G.P., Berger, J.L. and Bosson, M. (2008) 'Group assessment of learning potential of pupils in mainstream primary education and special education classes', *Journal of Cognitive Education and Psychology*, 7(1), pp. 43–69.

Kapantzoglou, M., Restrepo, M.A. and Thompson, M.S. (2012) 'Dynamic assessment of word learning skills: Identifying language impairment in bilingual children', *Language Speech and Hearing Services in Schools*, 43, pp. 81–96.

Larsen, J.A., and Nippold, M.A. (2007) 'Morphological analysis in school-age children: Dynamic assessment of a word learning strategy', *Language, Speech, and Hearing Services in Schools*, 38(3), pp. 201–212.

Lidz, C.S. (1991) *Practitioner's guide to dynamic assessment*, The Guilford Press, New York.

Lidz, C.S. (2003) *Early childhood assessment*, Wiley, Hoboken, NJ.

Peña, E.D., Gillam, R.B., Malek, M., Ruiz-Felter, R., Resendiz, M., Fiestas, C. and Sabel, T., 2006. 'Dynamic assessment of school-age children's narrative ability: An experimental investigation of classification accuracy'. *Journal of Speech, Language, and Hearing Research*, 49(5), pp. 1037–1056.

Olswang, L., and Bain, B. (1996) 'Assessment information for predicting upcoming change in language production', *Journal of Speech and Hearing Research*, 39(2), pp. 414–423.

Olswang, L., Bain, B. and Johnson, G. (1992) 'Using dynamic assessment with children with language disorders', Warren, S., and Reichle, J. (eds) *Causes and effects in communication and language intervention*, Paul H Brookes, Baltimore, MD.

Peña, E.D. (2000) 'Measurement of modifiability in children from culturally and linguistically diverse backgrounds', *Communication Disorders Quarterly*, 21(2), pp. 87–97.

Peña, E.D., and Iglesias, A. (1992) 'The application of dynamic methods to language assessment: A non-biased procedure', *The Journal of Special Education*, 26(3), pp. 269–280.

Peña, E.D., Iglesias, A. and Lidz, C.S. (2001) 'Reducing test bias through dynamic assessment of children's word learning ability', *American Journal of Speech-Language Pathology*, 10(2), pp. 138–154.

Ram, G., Marinellie, S.A., Benigno, J. and Mccarthy, J. (2013) 'Morphological analysis in context versus isolation: Use of a dynamic assessment task with school-age children', *Language, Speech, and Hearing Services in Schools*, 44, pp. 32–47.

Steele, S.C., and Watkins, R.V. (2010) 'Learning word meanings during reading by children with language learning disability and typically-developing peers', *Clinical Linguistics & Phonetics*, 24(7), pp. 520–539.

Vygotsky, L.S. (1986) *Thought and language*, MIT Press, Cambridge, MA.

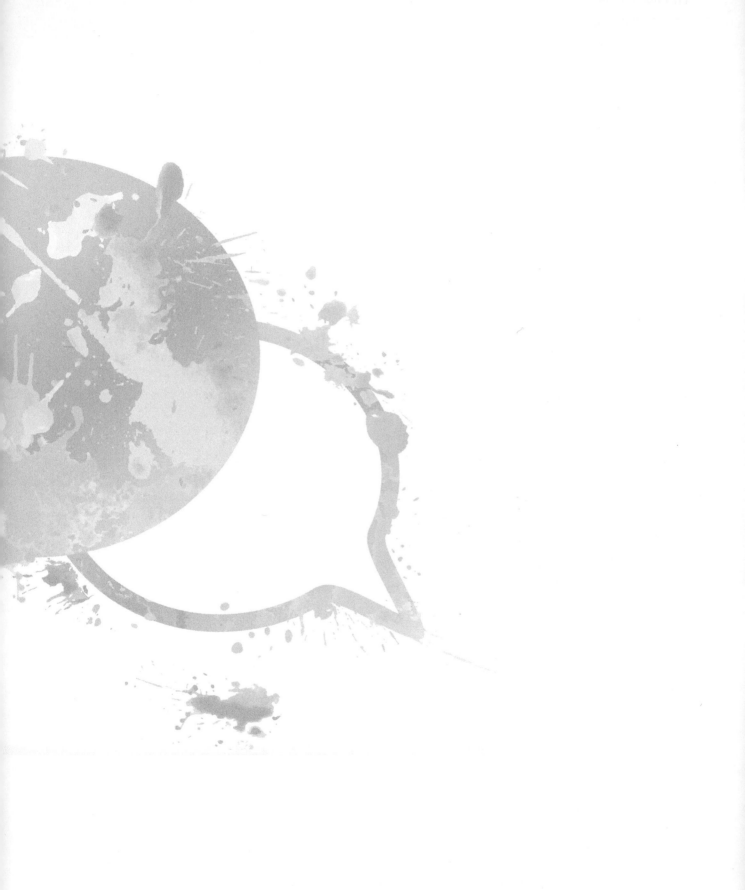

Chapter 3
How to do a DA

The range of tasks that can be addressed

    Phonology

    Morphology

    Word level

    Sentence level

    Narrative and discourse

The range of tasks that can be addressed

As we have seen from the review of previous research, a number of different areas of language have been addressed in DAs. There are also a number of different approaches to devising a DA. Any task can be adapted. Some lend themselves more easily to a breakdown of component skills, while others will need to be probed via 'clinical interview', which questions the responses elicited.

Using a modified linguistic/communication pyramid as a framework (Figure 3.1), in this section we will look in more detail at how to construct DAs for a range of tasks.

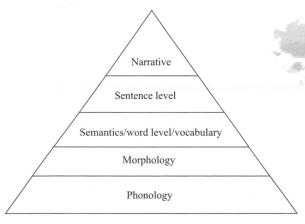

Figure 3.1 Levels of language framework for DAs

Phonology

Consider the following task:

Give two words that rhyme with 'round.'

There are many reasons why a child might struggle with an item like this. We need to ask what it is that would help the child succeed.

To do this, we need to analyse the task and break it down into all of its components.

1   Most broadly, does the child even know what he is supposed to do? Has he ever done this before, or is it completely strange? In other words, if we familiarised him with the task, would he then be able to do it?

2   Does he understand the instructions? *All* the vocabulary that is being used, including terms such as 'rhyme' and metalinguistic terms such as 'word', 'syllable' or 'sound?' What about 'beginning', 'end' or 'same'? We also need to monitor the grammar of the instruction and check that the child understands. If the instructions or items are written, we also need to check he can read them.

3   Only then do we get to the basic phonological skills. In order to generate a rhyme, you need to segment the word into onset and rime. Does the child know this? Can he do it? How can you explain it in terms he can understand?

4   Having segmented the word, can he hold the rime in his head and blend other consonants into the initial position? Does he know he has to do this? Can he hold it in his head or would written cues help? Would it be useful to have a written alphabet to work through?

5   Does the child recognise when a real word has been formed? Can he make the judgement between real and nonsense words?

6   When the child has generated one rhyming word, can he spontaneously repeat the process, or does he need scaffolding all over again? Can he transfer the cues to the next test item?

When you have thought through the task in detail like this, you are ready to construct a prompt hierarchy, or to begin to mediate to the child.

Consider the following tasks and carry out the same step-by-step analysis:

'Tell me the sound you hear at the beginning of the word *mouse*.'

Check that the child knows what you mean by a 'sound' and 'word', that he can segment the phonemes, that he understands the meaning of 'beginning' and that he understands that he must say the sound.

'Say the word *man*, but change the *m* for the sound *b*.

How might we construct a DA?

There are a number of options. At the outset, we might record the child's static performance on the test and find, for example, that he is unable to generate rhyming words. We might then demonstrate the task, emphasise the changing sounds, give examples and ask him to repeat models. At the end of this process, we would repeat the test and measure any improvement.

This *test-train-retest* would answer the questions posed in component 1. If the child is familiarised with the task, he may be able to do it, and the initial problem may have been one of lack of previous experience through poor stimulation or cultural difference, or he may not have understood what he needed to do and after some models can in fact complete the test.

If, however, the child still cannot do the task, we need to analyse, systematically, where the difficulty lies and what support is needed.

A hierarchy of prompts

The procedure of graduated prompting was introduced in Chapter 2. Prompts always need to be arranged into a consistent order, starting with the most broad and general (least helpful) and progressing, if needed, to more specific (more helpful) cues.

What kinds of prompts are 'broad and general'? Usually these are strategies of thinking and planning that are preparatory or generalisable to other tasks as well. Prepare the child by checking that he understands the task and that all the vocabulary is known and by teaching the necessary words that are not familiar. Does this enable him to do the task?

Generalisable cognitive skills are executive functions such as planning, hypothetical thinking and impulse control. Prompts at this level might be to facilitate the child to remember how he might have done a similar task before, or to plan and problem solve carefully.

When further prompts are required, because the child has not yet completed the task, more task-specific prompts are used. These depend on what the task is, so in the current example, that may be the segmenting of onset and rime, or general 'word play'. Writing words or letters may also be used.

Finally, and only if the child continues to struggle, the assessor may actually show the child how the answer is achieved.

So the prompt hierarchy might look like the one in Table 3.1:

Table 3.1 Prompt hierarchy for phonological analysis task. *Give two words that rhyme with 'round'*

	Prompt type	Example of prompt
1.	Instructions	Do you know what you have to do? Can you tell me?
2.	Preparation	Do you know what 'rhyme' means? Give me a 'word'. Do you know what a 'word' is? (Do man and can rhyme?)
3.	Cognitive strategies	Have you done this before? Do you remember what you did? What might you do first?
4.	Task specific	One part of the word needs to sound the same. Do you know which bit? Can you break the word up into parts? Use written cue *r/ound*. Can you change the first part?
5.	Item specific	OK, if we have 'r' and 'ound' and we take away the 'r', what do we have? Now put 's' in front. Does that make a real word? Do they rhyme? Now put k in front. Is that a real word?
6.	Transfer	Can you make another word? Is that right? How do you know?

The assessor can modify schemes like these to suit her purpose. Prompts may be more scripted and fixed if required to be standardised, or more questions may be inserted to probe further. A template for planning a prompt hierarchy for phonological tasks can be found in Appendix B02.

'Testing the Limits'

Alternatively, after the child answers the initial instruction, correctly or incorrectly, detailed feedback may be given.

"Yes, that's correct, *sound* does rhyme with *round*. How did you know? They both have the same sound at the end of the word, don't they? Both end in . . .? Yes, '*ound*'. What you have done is change the first part. What was that? The '*r*' to '*s*'. Round to sound. Can you hear how they sound the same? Like in a song, or a poem? Do 'round' and 'run' rhyme? Do they sound the same? What about round and found? And round and cound? Is that one right? Why not?"

Or,

"Why do you think 'mouse' is right? (This is not a rhetorical question; we actually want to find out what the child understands by the task and how he has determined his answer). Does 'mouse' rhyme with 'round'? What does 'rhyme' mean – do you know? (Explain what rhyme means). Now, let's see, do *round* and *mouse* sound the same? Is the end part the same? What is the end part of 'round?' Yes, '*ound*'. Can you think of another word with '*ound*?' "

When the next item is given, compare the child's response to the first item. Is it better? Has he retained the teaching? Give detailed feedback again and see if any parts have been learnt.

Mediated learning

Mediating the concept of rhyme generation to a young child would take a little longer than the other methods. We have seen that it is not a simple task; the rules of what constitutes a rhyme and the ability to segment words into constituent sounds are essential.

Many of the questions suggested earlier in the graded prompts and in the detailed feedback are mediational: they are probing to see what the child knows and facilitating him to problem solve. However, as we have seen, there are important components that make the teaching specifically mediational.

Does the child know why he is here?

Start with the explanation of what we are going to learn today, why it is important and what use it has. So we might say, "You know when you want to sing a song, or say a nursery rhyme? Like 'Hickory Dickory Dock?' Do you know that one? Can you say it for me/with me? Well, we are going to learn how songs and rhymes are made, so you can sing your own ones".

Or we might help an older child to understand that rhyming helps him learn how to read and spell some words.

When the child has grasped some of the applications, make sure he knows that you are going to help him to learn the skill. "So I am going to help you learn how to do this today. OK? And I need you to help me explain it to you, so you help me and tell me things. And then at the end, we will be able to say some really funny rhymes and sing some really funny songs, like 'Hickory Dickory Dock, the mouse ran up my sock (demonstrate)!' OK?"

Remember that a focus on rule-governed behaviour is one of the important cognitive skills to mediate. Make sure the child understands how rhyme works and does not generate random guesses.

Finally, make sure that you give plenty of praise and that it is specifically targeted. "Well done. You broke that word up perfectly. Now what do you need to do?" Or, "That's a really good try. I can see you are thinking about breaking up the word. Let's try and break it in a different place".

There are a number of different tasks under the umbrella of 'phonological processing' or PA skills, and they are needed and used by children in a wide age range. Which method of DA is used depends, as before, on the needs of the individual and the aims of the therapist, but in every instance, a detailed task analysis is an important place to start.

Morphology

The most common format for assessment of morphology in younger children is the procedure initiated by Berko in 1958, and still in use in various forms, using both real words and non-words (e.g. as 'word structure' testing in CELF-4, Semel, Wiig and Secord 2006)

Children are presented with real or nonsense items (Figure 3.2):

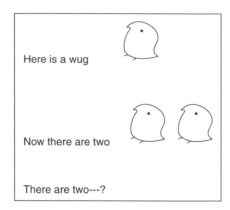

Here is a wug

Now there are two

There are two---?

Figure 3.2 Morphology test item (Berko 1958)

Once again, we need to analyse the task and consider the different reasons why a child might struggle with such a task. He may not be able to 'apply word structure rules' (CELF-4 Instruction Manual p.22 Objectives of the Word Structure subtest). Alternatively, he might not understand the task, might be confused by the pictures or nonsense words, might have a weak grasp of plurals, might not know the rule or might not be able to produce the required structure. A DA may be able to tease out which of these is the source of difficulty and identify what type of prompts are needed to facilitate the correct production.

In a test of morphology such as this, the items may address a range of morphological structures, such as plurals (both regular and irregular), auxiliaries, pronouns, comparatives and superlatives, third-person singular and past tenses (regular and irregular). The last two are known to be particularly problematic for children with language disorders. This means there is a lot of conceptual and grammatical knowledge, which may need to be assessed. A large number of test items or subtests, that each probe the child's grasp of a different grammatical structure, may be needed. A difficulty with appreciating and applying grammatical rules may underpin a number of different items, and if this were to be identified, it would help the therapist to determine more generalisable targets for intervention.

It is recommended, therefore, that a DA begin with the more general skills of problem solving, understanding of rules, phonological awareness (e.g. to add an [s] to the end of a word), before the task-specific aspects are examined. As noted earlier, this may be done with graded prompts, feedback or mediation. A template of graded prompts that may be adapted to DA of various morphological structures is contained in Appendix B03.

Mediational intervention, addressing cognitive skills and task awareness, would appear to be a practical way forward.

Test-teach-retest

A possible structure for a DA might be as follows:

- test – with a static morphological test;
- teach – possibly mediational intervention; and
- retest – with the same static assessment.

A published, standardised language test may be used as the pre-test. Caution should be taken when the test is repeated as a post-test after a very short interval, as standardised tests are not intended to be used in this way. However, from the theoretical standpoint of a DA, if a child is able to learn from doing a test once, and benefits from a 'practice effect', then he certainly has good potential to learn, and this is in itself informative.

A parallel form of the test, if one is available, is ideal. Alternatively, you can devise your own static pre-test.

The mediational intervention would target the principles of the task:

- What do you have to do?
- How do you know that?
- How can you do it?
- Look at this one (examples given). What has been done? Why did they do it like that? Why is that a good way?
- Can you do that with nonsense words? How do you know?
- Would a rule help us to know what to do?
- If we have that and that, then what rule can we make? Does it apply to this?
- Is that correct? How do you know?

> **Remember this?**
>
> *Ask process questions* (usually containing 'how').
>
> *Bridge to different applications.*
>
> *Challenge the child to justify his answers*, both right and wrong responses.
>
> *Teach about rules.*
>
> *Emphasise order, system, sequence and strategy.*
>
> *Create task-intrinsic motivation.*

To ensure the child understands the intentionality and meaning of the exercise he is doing, he might be asked the following:

"You know when some words have extra bits added onto the end, like an '-s' in 'book*s*', (use a written cue if appropriate)? Why do we do that? What does that '-s' mean? And when there is an '-s' like in 'run*s*', "the boy runs", does that also mean there are lots of them? What does it mean? What about '-ed' like in 'want*ed*'? Well these little endings tell us all kinds of extra things, and if we want people to understand exactly what we mean, then we need to make sure we have all these little parts exactly right. What might happen if your teacher asked you to get her the *book?* You'd get one, right? But what if she really wanted enough for the whole class? She'd have had to ask for . . .? So we are going to be looking at which little endings we need and what they all mean, and make sure that we use them correctly. OK?"

If this intervention (implemented optimally over two sessions) results in gains in the post-test, the prognosis for intervention would be positive. The teaching of separate grammatical rules for structures, if required, could then be a later stage.

The amount of improvement from the first test to retest would reflect the potential of the child to gain from the intervention and indicate whether the mediation addressed the child's difficulty on the test. In addition, we might look at how hard the therapist needed to work, or how much intervention or facilitation was needed in order for the child to improve from the first test to the post-test. This might also be an indication of the child's potential to learn.

An alternative approach to DA of morphology was taken by Larsen and Nippold (2007) in the Dynamic Assessment Task of Morphological Analysis (DATMA). The authors of this procedure set out to devise a DA to investigate whether school-age children could use morphological analysis to understand the meaning of complex morphological words such as they might find in a school curriculum. They also related this ability to the literacy skills of the children.

The procedure of graded prompts is shown in Table 3.2, adapted from Larsen and Nippold (2007 p. 204):

Table 3.2 Structure of the DATMA (Larsen and Nippold 2007)

	Prompt level	Example of prompt	Scoring
1	Open question, no cue	What does this word (X) mean?	5 points for correct response
2	Metacognitive reflection	How did you know?	to Prompt 1 and 2
3	Breaking down the task	Does X have smaller parts?	4
4	Item-specific support, morphological analysis	The parts are x and y. Now can you tell me what X means?	3
5	Item specific – context	Listen to the sentence and then tell me what X means.	2
6	Item specific – multiple choice	Which of these definitions explains X?	1
			0 for incorrect response

Ram *et al.* (2013) subsequently modified and tested the DATMA on a younger age group. A British adaptation that made use of vocabulary taken from the English national curriculum was piloted by Hasson *et al.* (2014). The procedure extended that of Larsen and Nippold, and is summarised in a flowchart, as seen in Appendix B04.

A hierarchy of prompts was used, which introduced the written word as an additional cue at each level. The prompts were qualitatively different, but progressively more supportive at each level. The prompts reflect techniques that may be used in intervention programmes, and the DA is therefore able to help the therapist determine what type of intervention strategies are useful for a given child. This is not unlike 'trial therapy', but the results are obtained within the single session that would usually be devoted to static assessment only.

Word level

Word knowledge, vocabulary or semantics is assessed in a number of different ways, tapping into both receptive and expressive skills.

Traditional assessments of receptive vocabulary frequently consist of a multiple-choice, picture-pointing task, such as the British Picture Vocabulary Scales (Dunn *et al.* 1997), Receptive One-Word Picture Vocabulary Test (Brownell 2010) or Peabody Picture Vocabulary Test (Dunn and Dunn 2007).

A dynamic version of this format was devised by Camilleri (Camilleri and Law 2007) to assess the potential for 'fast mapping' in preschool children. Fast mapping is the ability to establish an immediate link between a word and its referent on first or with little exposure to the word in the presence of the object (Carey, 1978, cited by Camilleri and Law 2007). In this DA procedure, prompts were given to assist the child to identify the named picture using the process of elimination of known words, as shown in Table 3.3, adapted from Camilleri and Law (2007).

Table 3.3 Structure of the DA of vocabulary (Camilleri and Law 2007)

	STAGE	PROCEDURE	SCORE
1	Static pre-test	BPVS	
2	Selection of target materials	Six items (preferably three nouns, three verbs) that the child did not know in the static pre-test	
3	Interactive phase 1 Independent problem solving	Present three cards, two known and one previously unknown. Ask child to find target (unknown) item	If correct score 3

(*Continued*)

Table 3.3 (Continued)

	STAGE	PROCEDURE	SCORE
4	Phase 2: 'Implicit identification'	If child was incorrect in phase 1, ask him to find the two (familiar) distractor items	Score 2
5	Phase 3: 'Explicit identification'	If child is still incorrect, ask child to identify distractors and then turn them face down, leaving target only	Score 1
6	Expressive task 1	Ask child which item he would like to post in the box	Number of target items named
7	Retention of meaning	Child asked to point to each of three previously targeted items	Number of items retained
8	Expressive task 2	Second opportunity to name the newly learnt items	Number of target items named
9	Receptive post-test	Child asked to point to all six items as they were named. No feedback given until all six are completed	Number of items retained

The procedure was shown to differentiate children referred to speech and language therapists from those with no identified concerns, and it was effective in both monolingual and bilingual children. It was subsequently also shown to increase the predictive value of the static assessment in low-scoring children. It is particularly useful in young children, as it has a lower demand on verbal skills and demonstrates how the stimulability of very young children may be probed in the assessment.

Camilleri further developed the Dynamic Assessment of Word Learning (Camilleri and Botting 2013), which aimed to assess vocabulary learning in a more naturalistic context, approximating a child's everyday learning of vocabulary at school. Children who did not spontaneously name a target object when describing a complex picture were prompted to establish word-referent matches. The first cue had the word embedded within three sentences about the picture. The next more specific cue described the meaning of the target word, followed by signalling it in the picture and finally explicit pointing and identification. At each level, the child's ability to identify the target in two instances in the picture was taken as grasping semantic content.

Test-mediate-retest

Peña and Gillam (2000) devised an assessment of vocabulary for preschool children from diverse linguistic and cultural backgrounds. The procedure used the Expressive One-Word Picture

Vocabulary Test (EOWPVT-R, Gardner 1979, cited in Peña and Gillam 2000) as a static pre- and post-test measure, but modified the administration to include a minimum of 30 items and permitted responses in more than one language. Two sessions of mediated intervention focused on the concept of 'special names' or the use of precise vocabulary. Designated materials were used to address selected categories of vocabulary, and mediation was scripted for consistency. The child's responses to mediation and cognitive abilities were noted.

Pre-post-test scores were used as well as qualitative changes to response types. The examiner also judged child responsivity and examiner effort. These observations have been shown to be good indicators of ability. Finally, the ability of the child to transfer his learning to new items was observed. This method of DA of vocabulary is especially useful for bilingual children who are credited for knowledge in a different language and who perform in qualitatively different ways than children with language disorders.

Clinical interviewing and feedback

In these procedures, described by Peña (2001), enhanced techniques of assessment similar to those used before were used to probe the word knowledge of children from different linguistic and cultural backgrounds whose performances on standardised tests may have been affected by a range of factors owing to cultural experiences and expectations.

In the feedback condition, children's naming responses were met with positive feedback, "Good. You gave me a special name for that", or with further probes such as "You've told me what it does, now can you think of a special name for it?", or "Do you know another name?" In this way, the assessor gauged semantic organisation abilities and lexical retrieval, as well as semantic and conceptual knowledge, and the children achieved higher scores. Case comparison revealed that greater insight into a child's semantic development was enabled.

However, while face validity of the procedure is high, Peña stresses that reliability is not established, and clinicians should follow procedures to increase reliability:

- Plan the feedback beforehand.
- Think about the goal for feedback.
- Consider possible child responses and plan follow-up questions.
- Keep careful notes of the feedback or instructions given.
- Be consistent in the use of techniques.
- Review notes and audiotapes to clarify techniques used.

And finally, remember that a lack of improvement through feedback does not automatically signal language impairment, and other facilitations might be useful.

In the clinical interview situation, further questioning is used as well as feedback. Like the procedure described earlier, it is important to structure the interview questions, as described by Ginsburg (1997, cited by Peña 2001).

1   Analyse the child's *competence* in the key abilities, his level of skill or knowledge.

2   *Explore* the child's problem solving, strategies and approaches by probing with further questions that reveal concept organisation and links between concepts.

3   Form *hypotheses* about why the child uses certain strategies and skills, and explore these hypotheses.

4   Formulate a *theory* about the child's competence.

(Ginsburg 1997, cited by Peña 2001)

Peña then designed a clinical interview to investigate semantic knowledge and specified the targets of part-whole relationships, description of functions, linguistic concepts, similarities and differences, categorisations and analogies. The interview was embedded in a play activity based on a house puzzle (Table 3.4).

Table 3.4 Clinical interview of semantic knowledge (Peña 2001)

Semantic area	Initial questions	Possible follow-up
Part-whole	What parts does a house have?	What does the word 'parts' mean? Draw a house based on the child's directions, examine together and discuss what parts are still needed. Ask the child how he knew this.
Functions	What is a door for? What do windows do?	Do most things have uses? How do you know? What would happen if you didn't have a door?
Linguistic concepts	How many windows are there? What colour do you want to use to colour the house? Let's see what shapes are in the house. Can you tell me?	How did you figure out that number? Hand child wrong colour crayon and observe reaction. How do you know it's a square not a triangle? What are shapes? Colours? Numbers?
Similarities and differences	How are doors and windows similar? How are they different?	What does similar mean? Difference? How do you figure out similarities and differences?

Semantic area	Initial questions	Possible follow-up
Categorisations	What kinds of things are in the house?	Could a correct/incorrect item go in the house? Why/Why not?
	What foods do you think could be in the fridge?	How do you figure that out?
	What do you think is in the garage?	What's a category? How do you know what things go together in a category?
Analogies (older children only)	Garage is to large as bathroom is to?	How did you get that answer? Is a garage big or little? Can you think of another word for big? What about a bathroom? Is it big or little?

Reprinted with permission. Peña E. D. (2001) 'Assessment of Semantic Knowledge: Use of Feedback and Clinical Interviewing', *Seminars in Speech and Language*, 22(1), pp 51–63.

These tasks are familiar components of static language assessments and subtests. Include whichever aspects you are trying to assess, for example picture naming, word associations etc., or combine them as in this example. Standardised tests may be used as the baseline or pre-test for an intervention such as this, but remember not to teach to the items of a standardised test, or you will invalidate it for future use.

Again, while the evidence for the procedure is case based, Peña emphasises the need for planning, consistency and record keeping in the assessment. Repeat the procedure using a different stimulus to see whether responses are consistent or improvement has been facilitated. As before, there is the option to add more facilitations or mediations to the procedure as further follow-up prompts, and in some tasks, such as "How do x and y go together?", word definitions or "name as many animals as you can in one minute", more in-depth mediation would seem to be a logical step.

Adaptations of Peña's clinical interview technique may be used for a range of both receptive and expressive vocabulary or word-knowledge tasks. Subtests of standardised tests such as the CELF-4 (Semel, Wiig, and Secord 2006) expressive vocabulary, word classes and word definitions may be used as baseline pre-tests, but the items of these tests should *never* be used for mediation in order not to invalidate further use of the test. Instead, devise and use similar items to those in the test to probe responses and ask, "Why do you call it that?", "What is another name for that?" and other probing questions such as those used by Peña above.

Expressive naming tests always require judgements about the acceptability of responses, which are slightly subjective, so standardised normative tests are often not the best way to approach the assessment of a child's expressive naming skills. Qualitative dynamic methods may be seen to be more functional assessments of vocabulary.

Sentence level

There are several assessments of sentence-level receptive language, which tap into the complex semantic and syntactic relationships of words in a sentence. These, like the assessments of words and semantic relationships addressed earlier, are probably most informatively probed by clinical interview and mediation techniques.

Expressive sentence formulation is more difficult to assess in a standardised form, as the range of acceptable answers is necessarily vast. Tightly controlled tasks such as sentence repetition are very useful in the static form. Language sampling techniques, such as Language Assessment, Remediation and Screening Procedure (Crystal, Fletcher and Garman 1976), are not formal or norm referenced tests, and as such, the interactive, conversational sampling of language can include a range of probing questions. The responses to these can be analysed both in terms of their grammatical structure and the information that they yield. They also provide opportunities for spontaneous prompting – for example, to see whether an individual is able to complete an unfinished sentence, make grammatical judgements and self-correct, or imitate a given structure. The skilled mediator would be able to facilitate improved conversational interaction from her client and also glean evaluative information about the client's communication.

There are few DAs that address expressive formulation of sentences. An early study by Hasson (2005) illustrates a test-mediate-retest approach to the assessment of receptive and expressive language skills, in a task based on the format of the Renfrew Action Picture Test (RAPT, Renfrew 1988). The RAPT is an expressive test of language that requires children aged three to eight to answer a question based on a given picture. The response is scored both on the information it contains and the grammatical structure of the utterance.

The dynamic version offered four sessions of mediated intervention in which all aspects of the task were addressed – for example, understanding of the task, recognition of the elements of the picture and vocabulary for items in the picture, understanding of the grammar of the test question and formulation of the response. The qualitative pre-test to post-test changes were analysed to gain understanding of the strengths and needs of each child, and to make recommendations for their future intervention.

The four mediated intervention sessions made use of task materials parallel to those of the RAPT – the same in structure, but without using the materials of the RAPT in order not to teach the test. The grammatical structures were the same, but content differed, and the concepts contained in the content were therefore different. In one example, the picture showed a father turning off the light in a child's room with the child in bed. One child was unable to grasp the events represented and the idea that the light would be turned off as the child went to sleep. Difficulties with sequences, routines and conceptual understanding contributed to this child's linguistic difficulties.

Pictures and prompt questions were presented. If the child struggled, a pre-planned sequence of prompts was used, gradually increasing the directions given to the child (see Table 3.5). The questions and further prompts were rated according to Feuerstein's RMI (Feuerstein *et al.* 2002) (See Appendix B01) so that at the end of the process, a clear idea had been obtained of the nature and intensity of intervention required to enable the child to manage a task of this type.

Table 3.5 Test protocol for DA of language (Hasson 2005)

SUMMARY OF PROCEDURE:

1 TEST PHASE

Original standardised version of test (RAPT)

2 TRAINING PHASE

  Additional materials – pictures with prompts illustrating sentences similar in structure to those targeted in the test

Present picture and ask question.

Prompt using the following, in given sequence:

  1 Specific elicitation questions

  - What can you see in the picture?
  - What is happening here?
  - Who is this? (and this?)
  - What is he/what are they doing?
  - What (object) is this?
  - What was the question?
  - What did they ask you to look for?
  - Which parts of the picture tell us that?
  - What should we tell them first? And then?
  - Shall we practice the answer?
  - Do we need to say this?

(Continued)

Table 3.5 (Continued)

---

2 **Question broken into parts**

3 **Cloze prompts**

4 **Choices**

5 **Direct modelling and request for imitation**

Elicit second attempt at answer.

Then show next picture and repeat.

3 RETEST PHASE

Repeat original test.

Standardised version of test

4 EVALUATE CHANGE

Responses obtained by the children during the intervention were recorded and transcribed.

In addition, the relevant cognitive functions from the range of functions identified by Feuerstein *et al.* (2002) were considered during the mediation process and the child rated on a five-point scale for the quality of the cognitive process (see Appendix B05).

The study revealed that children who all performed at the lowest level on the static form of the RAPT were widely differentiated by the DA procedure, according to their responses, needs and rates of improvement. The RMI levels needed to elicit responses and the nature of the improved responses were most informative.

A further study, based on a similar methodology (Hasson and Botting 2010), became a pilot study for the DASS, which will be described in Chapter 5. The task was based on the Sentence Assembly subtest of the CELF-3 (UK) (Semel, Wiig and Secord 1987), but as in the previous task, the items of the CELF subtest were not used for training. Instead, 48 similar items were devised, carefully arranged according to grammatical structure and complexity, and the children worked through these with supportive mediation over three sessions. The children were scored according to their improvement from the pre-test to the post-test and the level of prompting on the RMI scale (Feuerstein *et al.* 2002). In addition, behavioural observations were recorded. Three children aged 11–12 years, all with previously identified language disorders, participated in the study. The procedure, and primarily the RMI and behavioural observations, was shown to distinguish three different presentations and indicate clinically useful profiles for the three children, all of whom had similar results on static standardised tests.

Addressing a simpler level of sentence formulation, Bain and Olswang (1995) devised a procedure for prompting preschool children to join words into two-word utterances (previously mentioned in Chapter 2). The procedure adapted a prompt hierarchy to be suitable for very young children and involved the examiner manipulating objects while providing children with a hierarchy of verbal cues and prompts, as follows in Table 3.6:

Table 3.6 Prompt structure for DA of two-word utterances

	Prompt type	Example
1	General Statement	Look here.
2	Elicitation Statement	What is this?
3	Sentence Completion	The man is. . .?
4	Indirect Model	Man is walking. What is he doing?
5	Direct Model	The man is walking.
6	Direct Model + Elicitation	Say, the man is walking.

Adapted from Bain and Olswang (1995).

This procedure informed the brief intervention included in the sentence component of the DAPPLE (Hasson, Dodd and Botting 2012).

Narrative and discourse

Four publications that employ DA methods and deal with discourse or story-level texts are included here as examples of the methods that may be used.

Peña and Gillam (2000) first used a test-mediate-retest structure in which children were required to tell and retell stories based on a large and interesting picture. Narratives were rated for elements of story structure and content. Two 20-minute sessions of mediated intervention addressed story structure.

Miller, Gillam and Peña (2001) subsequently published the *Dynamic Assessment of Narrative*, which is one of the few published DAs of language. The task retained the test-teach-retest structure, with two sessions of mediational intervention in the teach phase. The targets of the intervention were individually selected for the children and addressed their ability to retell a story from a wordless picture book. Aspects of story construction and the inclusion of essential elements were addressed. A sample of the mediation used by the authors is reprinted in Appendix B06.

A further study carried out by Elleman *et al.* (2011) addressed the ability of children to draw inferences from story information in order to identify children at risk for developing reading difficulties because of poor comprehension. The procedure was essentially a graduated prompt procedure with seven short passages on familiar topics, which were read aloud to the children.

Children were scored on three open-ended questions for each story, one requiring inference about story setting and the other two requiring causal inferences.

The procedure consisted of the following:

1   A pre-test story with no feedback given

2   A lesson about being a 'reading detective' using practice story 2

3   The 'dynamic phase' of three stories with prompting until correct; five levels of prompting were used

4   A post-test story with no feedback given

5   A transfer story with low cohesion and no feedback

6   A transfer-expository text with no feedback

Elleman found that the number of prompts and total DA scores strongly correlated with reading in a static test of passage comprehension. The DA, therefore, measures a similar construct to reading comprehension, but more than word identification or vocabulary measures. Furthermore, the DA enabled identification of more intra-individual differences in reading abilities.

One further procedure documented by Peña and Gillam (2000) pertains to 'explanatory discourse' and is most useful with older children. In this example, the pre-and post-test static tests are first all the even items and then all the odd-numbered items from the Test of Problem Solving (TOPS Zachman *et al.* 1994, cited in Peña and Gillam 2000). The discussion around the given situations lends itself well to mediation of problem identification and problem-solving strategies, planning and delivery of responses. Peña and Gillam were able to score the improvement on the test, as well as the syntax used in responses, and rate the examiner effort required to elicit changes.

The broad scope of narrative or discourse means that task analyses may be complex, or that several different aspects may be addressed separately. For example, the mediational programme used by Peña and Gillam focuses on story structure, while the programme by Elleman addresses inference. The static tests of narrative that are available are similarly based on different aspects of the task, the Bus Story Test (Renfrew 2010) on inclusion of the main elements of content of the story and the grammar used in retelling, while the Expression, Reception and Recall of Narrative Instrument (ERRNI) (Bishop 2004) scores literal and inferential comprehension as well as story recall. Dynamic tasks may use these static tests as pre- and post-test measures and devise interventions or mediations to assess readiness to improve in ways that the tests might measure.

In summary, when devising a DA, it is important to analyse the task at hand carefully and consider what the individual is required to know and to do in order to complete the task

Different methods of DA can be used, depending on the task, but DAs can be devised to probe an individual's learning of a range of linguistic structures.

References

Bain, B.A., and Olswang, L. (1995) 'Examining readiness for learning two-word utterances by children with specific expressive language impairment: Dynamic assessment validation', *American Journal of Speech-Language Pathology*, 4, pp. 81–91.

Berko, J. (1958) 'The child's learning of English morphology', *Word*, 14(2–3), pp. 150–177.

Bishop, D. (2004) *Expression, reception and recall of narrative instrument (ERRNI)*, Pearson Clinical, Oxford.

Brownell, R. (2010) *Receptive and expressive one-word picture vocabulary tests*, 4th Edn, Pearson Clinical, Oxford.

Camilleri, B., and Botting, N. (2013) 'Beyond static assessment of children's receptive vocabulary: The dynamic assessment of word learning', *International Journal of Language and Communication Disorders*, 48(5), pp. 565–581.

Camilleri, B., and Law, J. (2007) 'Assessing children referred to speech and language therapy: Static and dynamic assessment of receptive vocabulary', *International Journal of Speech-Language Pathology*, 9(4), pp. 312–322.

Crystal, D., Fletcher, P. and Garman, M. (1976) *The grammatical analysis of language disability: A procedure for assessment and remediation*, Edward Arnold, London.

Dunn, D.M., and Dunn, L.M. (2007) *Peabody picture vocabulary test*, 4th edn, Pearson Clinical, Oxford.

Dunn, L.M., Dunn, D.M., Whetton, C. and Burley, J. (1997) *The British picture vocabulary scale II*, 2nd edn, NFER Nelson, Berkshire.

Elleman, A.M., Compton, D.L., Fuchs, D., Fuchs, L.S. and Bouton, B. (2011) 'Exploring dynamic assessment as a means of identifying children at risk of developing comprehension difficulties', *Journal of Learning Disabilities*, 44(4), pp. 348–357.

Feuerstein, R., Feuerstein, R.S., Falik, L.H. and Rand, Y. (2002) *The dynamic assessment of cognitive modifiability: The learning propensity assessment device: Theory, instruments and techniques*, ICELP Press, Jerusalem.

Hasson, N. (2005) *The use of dynamic methods of language assessment in language impaired children*. Poster presented to IACEP conference, Durham.

Hasson, N., and Botting, N. (2010) 'Dynamic assessment of children with language impairments: A pilot study', *Child Language Teaching and Therapy*, 26(3), pp. 249–272.

Hasson, N., Dodd, B. and Botting, N. (2012) 'Dynamic Assessment of Sentence Structure (DASS): Design and evaluation of a novel procedure for assessment of syntax in children with language impairments', *International Journal of Language and Communication Disorders*, 47(3), pp. 285–299.

Hasson, N., Nash, L., Cubie, B., Kessie, A. and Marshall, C. (2014) *Dynamic assessment of morphological analysis: A UK based study.* Poster presented to RCSLT Conference, University of Leeds.

Larsen, J.A., and Nippold, M.A. (2007) 'Morphological analysis in school-age children: Dynamic assessment of a word learning strategy', *Language, Speech, and Hearing Services in Schools*, 38(3), pp. 201–212.

Miller, L., Gillam, R.B. and Peña, E.D. (2001) *Dynamic assessment and intervention: Improving children's narrative abilities*, Pro-Ed, Austin, TX.

Peña, E.D. (2001) 'Assessment of semantic knowledge: Use of feedback and clinical interviewing', *Seminars in Speech and Language*, 22(1), pp. 51–63.

Peña, E.D., and Gillam, R.B. (2000) 'Dynamic assessment of children referred for speech and language evaluations', Lidz, C.S., and Elliott, J. (eds) *Dynamic assessment: Prevailing models and applications*, Elsevier Science, Amsterdam.

Ram, G., Marinellie, S.A., Benigno, J. and McCarthy, J. (2013) 'Morphological analysis in context versus isolation: Use of a dynamic assessment task with school-age children', *Language, Speech, and Hearing Services in Schools*, 44, pp. 32–47.

Renfrew, C. (1988) *The Renfrew action picture test*, Winslow Press, Bicester.

Renfrew, C. (2010) *The bus story (Revised)*, Speechmark, Abingdon.

Semel, E., Wiig, E.H. and Secord, W. (1987) *Clinical evaluation of language fundamentals*, 3rd edn, The Psychological Corporation, London.

Semel, E., Wiig, E.H. and Secord, W. (2006) *Clinical evaluation of language fundamentals*, 4th edn, Pearson, Oxford.

Chapter 4
Scoring

Scoring of prompt hierarchies

Scoring of mediation

Ratings of modifiability

We have seen the range of different methodologies of DA and the decisions regarding test structure that need to be made when setting up a dynamic test procedure. Following on from this there will be decisions regarding the measurements to be made and the scores which will be used.

Guthke, Beckmann and Dobat (1997 p. 24) summarised the process as follows:

Options one has when using dynamic testing:

1 One test session only or use of a pre-post-test design on the basis of one or several post-tests

2 Determining the number and kind(s) of prompts, additional items and feedback information, or determination of the learning gained in a post-test compared with the pre-test

3 Use of difference scores (pre-test, post-test, absolute or relative scores) or post-test scores, use of goal attainment or learning success criteria

4 Determining learning gains only quantitatively or determination of qualitative 'types of change'

5 Assessing only learning gains or 'learning processes'

We will look at some of these options in more detail.

Scoring of prompt hierarchies

The intention of the authors of this methodology was that scoring should be enabled by directly counting the number of prompts or cues delivered. To this end, cognitive psychologists and EPs devised assessments that can be delivered electronically, which enables precise measurement and counting of prompts – for example, the Computer Assisted Intelligence Learning Tests Battery (Guthke, Beckmann and Dobat 1997).

Fixed-cue hierarchies, such as the examples given for the DATMA and adaptations of that measure for assessment of morphological awareness (Larsen and Nippold 2007; Ram *et al.* 2013; Hasson *et al.* 2014) (see Chapter 3) permit standardised counts of the cues and reliable scoring.

However, in many instances, the learning process is more complicated than the prompt structure would capture. Resing (1997) described the steps used in the training procedure of a test-train-retest DA of children's analogical reasoning. The prompts were classified into metacognitive or cognitive, and the necessary training levels were described. The procedure was limited to seven steps, but it can be seen that within some of the steps, additional training cues are given (page 74). The study found that the number of hints required (between one and seven for each trial), as well as post-test scores, were good predictors of school performance.

Subsequently, Resing *et al.* (2009) found that they needed to also count the number and type of attempts the children made to solve the task and classify their use of strategies.

As an example of the method for counting the levels of prompts, let us take another look at the proposed structure for prompting in a phonological task that was given in Chapter 3.

Give two words that rhyme with 'round'

Prompt type	Example of prompt
Instructions	Do you know what you have to do?
	Can you tell me?
Preparation	Do you know what 'rhyme' means?
	Do you know what a 'word' is?
	(Do man and can rhyme?)
Cognitive strategies	Have you done this before?
	Do you remember what you did?
	What might you do first?
Task specific	One part of the word needs to sound the same. Do you know which bit?
	Can you break the word up into parts?
	Use written cue *r/ound*.
	Can you change the first part?
Item specific	OK, if we have 'r' and 'ound' and we take away the 'r', what do we have?
	Now put 's' in front.
	Does that make a real word?
	Do they rhyme?
	Now put k in front. Is that a real word?

Prompt type	Example of prompt
Transfer	Can you make another word?
	Is that right?
	How do you know?

It is clear that within each of the 'prompt-type' bands, there are several questions.

There are two options for scoring: either a count of each individual prompt question or a record of the level of prompt required. As always, the choice might rest on the individual child and the assessor's aims for the assessment.

In order to carry out a count of every individual prompt question, the assessor would need to record the session and transcribe the interaction verbatim. This will reveal detailed information about a child's ability to grasp the task, process the phonology and use the different facilitations to succeed in the task. The amount of prompting, or facilitation that the assessor needs to contribute, is a measure of the child's learning needs. Scores on successive items will indicate his retention and transfer of strategies learnt from the intervention. Qualitative examination of the cues that the child found helpful suggests directions for future intervention strategies.

The difficulty with counting every cue is that many of the assessor's cues are not strictly necessary, but, as in the example noted earlier and the transcription that follows, serve the purposes of maintaining conversation and contributing mediation. Mediational utterances give feedback and reinforcement (mediation of competence), set out the task (intentionality), reinforce rules (rule-governed behaviour) and encourage the child to reflect (challenge). Planning to count each cue would mean restricting the assessor's input to the strictly facilitative cues. An alternative measure might be to count how many attempts the child makes before additional cues are added. Again, it would be necessary to be very consistent about how many times the child is permitted to make an attempt before an additional cue is given.

Counting and recording the level of prompting required in order for the child to succeed in the task, is quicker and can be carried out while the assessment progresses When the child succeeds in giving the target response, the level that has been reached is noted, that is, there is a score between one and five, relating to the prompt level in the diagram. This is useful, as several items can be administered and a tally of the scores retained so that improvement from item to item is immediately visible. A total score is also useful if management decisions or priorities for intervention need to be determined immediately after the assessment. Limitations of this method are that the nature of prompts in each level need to be very clearly defined and consistently implemented.

Both methods can, of course, be employed simultaneously by recording the levels on paper during the assessment and transcribing a full audio or video recording afterwards to obtain detailed information. An illustration of this procedure, taken from the author's research into the DASS, is provided next. The task was not phonological, but a sentence assembly task, which will be fully described in Chapter 5, as will the hierarchical scoring.

Utterance No.	Speaker		Notes
1	N (assessor)	Do you know what you have to do?	Metacognitive cue. Level 1
2	C (Child)	Man is the wall painting my	Reading words as they appear on the card
3	C	That's very good reading. What do you have to do with that, do you think?	Feedback Metacognitive cue
4	C	You have to swap them around.	
5	N	That's right. To make what?	
6	C	To make a sentence.	Metalinguistic knowledge
7	N	A proper sentence, well done. So can you do that one?	Feedback
8	C	Yes.	
9	N	OK. You have a try.	
10	C	My. . .	
11	N	OK. We are going to do these together so if you can't do it, you tell me and I'll help you. OK?	Mediation of intentionality
12	C	My. . . man. . . is. . . painting. . . my wall!	
13	N	Very good! Did you use up all the words?	Prompt for reflection
14	C	(Head nods)	
15	N	So say it again for me.	
16	C	The man (N – Yes) is painting my wall.	SCORE 1
17	N	Well done. I wasn't sure if you had used 'the', but you did. Very good. Is that right? Is that a good sentence do you think?	Feedback

Prompt for reflection |
| 18 | C | Yes. | |
| 19 | N | How do you know? | Prompt for metacognitive reflection |

Utterance No.	Speaker		Notes
20	C	Because I said . . . the man	
21	N	And you used up all the words. We have to use all the words, don't we?	Reinforcing rules
22	C	Yes.	
23	N	OK. And now can you make another one? Another sentence with the same words? OK?	
24	C	My wall . . . is painting . . . the man!	Aware of absurdity
25	N	(Laughs) Can the wall paint the man?	
26	C	The man is . . . ? (big sigh)	
27	N	OK, don't worry. I'm going to help you. We have to start with something different.	Level 3 cue
28	C	Right. Is . . . the man . . . painting my wall?	SCORE 3
29	N	Very good! How did you know which one to start with?	Prompt for reflection
30	C	I start the man cos he's the peo – par, par . . . man.	
31	N	Person	
32	N	And that time you started with 'is'. How did you know you had to start with 'is'?	
33	C	Because the . . . and I said the is wall paint my man. What I do? Man painting the wall!	
34	N	Very good, and that time you started with 'is' and you said, "Is the man painting my wall?"	Feedback
35	N	What kind of sentence is that?	
36	C	Er . . .	
37	N	Asking a . . . ?	
38	C	Question	Metalinguistic knowledge

(*Continued*)

(Continued)

Utterance No.	Speaker		Notes
39	N	Good girl, yes. That was a good way of doing it wasn't it, asking a question?	
40	C	Yes. I wanted a question.	
41	N	You wanted a question, so you started with . . . ? Is.	
42	C	Yes.	
43	N	That's a very good way of doing it.	
	N	OK (presents card #2).	
44	C	Billy . . .	
45	N	Do you know that word?	Level 2 cue
46	C	Billy scored.	
47	N	Hang on – that word – goal.	
48	C	Goal. Billy scored . . . is . . . Billy scored is . . . scored is . . . scored . . . is going a. . . That's not right!	
49	N	That's not right, is it? So what are you going to do?	Level 2 cue
50	C	Billy is scored. . . going . . . Billy scored. . . Billy scored is . . . to (sighs).	
51	N	Oh, tricky isn't it? Billy is a good place to start. After Billy, what are we looking for?	Level 4 cue
52	C	Billy . . . going . . . to score is score.	
53	N	OK, you're getting there. We had Billy going to score . . . What's he going to score?	Level 5 cue
54	C	Um, don't know.	
55	N	What's this word?	
56	C	Goal.	
57	N	Goal, yes. What's Billy going to score?	Level 5 cue
58	C	A goal.	

Utterance No.	Speaker		Notes
59	N	A goal, that's right. He might be playing football right? OK, so let's make sure you've used up all the words.	Reinforcing rules
60	C	Billy scored.	
61	N	No, Billy . . .	
62	C	Billy scored . . .	
63	N	No, Billy is . . .	Level 5 cue
64	C	Billy is going to scored . . . going to score a . . . nah . . . a goal (with N pointing to each word).	SCORE 5
65	N	Billy is going to score a goal. Got it? Tricky one isn't it? Yeah. He's going to score a goal.	
66	N	What do you have to do now? We have to make another one, don't we?	
67	C	No!	
68	N	Yes we do. You know how to make another one; you made one before. So how do we do it? You know how to do it; you did it before	Level 2 cue
69	C	Billy is . . .	
70	N	What do we have to do to make another one? You have to.	
71	C	Start!	
72	N	Yes, what are we going to start with?	Level 3 cue
73	C	A person!	
74	N	We always start with a person – but now we're going to make something different so we need to start with something different	Level 3 cue

(*Continued*)

(Continued)

Utterance No.	Speaker		Notes
75	C	Is . . . Billy . . . scored . . . going to . . .	
76	N	Yes, good. Is Billy going to. . .	Level 5 cue
77	C	Score a ma . . . a goal (goal – said simultaneously with N)	SCORE 5
78	N	Is that a good one?	Prompt for reflection
79	C	Yeah.	
80	N	Is it right? How do you know it's right?	Prompt for reflection
81	C	Because . . . because some . . .	
82	N	Does it make sense?	Reinforcing rules
83	C	Yes. Makes sense.	
84	N	It makes sense. Did you use up all the words?	Prompt for reflection
85	C	Yes.	
86	N	You did. Wait. You were very good; you started with 'is Billy'. How did you remember to do that?	Reinforcing rules. Prompt for reflection
87	C	Because, I *rembered*.	Metacognitive awareness
88	N	You remembered? Where did you remember from?	
89	C	You said.	
90	N	I said? Because we did it on the one before and you remembered?	
91	C	Yes.	
92	N	Well, that's very clever to remember what you did before and then do it again.	Reinforcing metacognitive strategy
93	C	Yeah (happy).	

The level of the prompts can be noted immediately, while at the same time a great deal of qualitative information is also to be gained from analysis of the transcription. For example, it is noticeable that the child's metacognitive and metalinguistic awareness are relatively good in the presence of very poor expressive language skills. This will be explored further in Chapter 6.

Scoring of mediation

Mediational interventions are typically part of the test-teach-retest process. These methods are scored by comparison of the pre- and post-test scores, which are static procedures, and therefore have standardised scoring.

The improvement from pre- to post-test is known as the 'gain score' and represents how much an individual is able to improve after a short period of intervention; in other words, his zone of proximal development. There is some controversy, however, about the statistical properties of gain scores, related first to practice effects (Swanson and Lussier 2001) and second to the need to account for pre-test performance (Carlson and Wiedl 1978; Embretson 1987). For these reasons, many researchers advocate the use of pre-test scores, post-test scores and 'post-test adjusted for pre-test level' as outcome variables. However, for clinical purposes, rather than research, an individual's pre-test and gain scores are informative. Considering the numerical scores on these static tests does, however, overlook the wealth of additional qualitative information that is available from the DA.

The additional information is determined by close examination of the content of the training phase. The process of mediation is necessarily individualised and adapted to the individual's responses, and therefore unscripted. It is also, therefore, less easy to score quantitatively.

The 'level of cues' described earlier is consistent with the theory of mediational intervention and based on the scoring protocol devised by Feuerstein *et al.* (2002) – namely, the RMI. As discussed in Chapter 2, the RMI is a set of descriptors capturing both the assessor's inputs and the testee's responses (see Appendix B01). Mediational interventions can then be quantitatively scored using this measure of the intervention.

In an attempt to determine the degree to which any interaction could be characterised as mediational, Lidz (1991) developed the Mediated Learning Experience Rating Scale. Lidz operationally defined the essential components of mediational interaction, previously described by Feuerstein and his colleagues, and rated each one on a scale of 0–3, according to whether they were delivered by the mediator. The examiner (or assessor, therapist or parent) was scored between 0 and 3 for each of 12 mediational characteristics:

0 = not in evidence

1 = clear, but not elaborated reference

2 = elaborated reference

3 = elaborated + a description for each behaviour of what the highest level of achievement would be

(Lidz 1991 p. 106–111)

The interested reader is referred to Lidz (1991 or 2003) for a detailed description of the scale, which is also reproduced in Appendix B07.

Lidz (1991) notes that the MLE Rating Scale focuses entirely on the mediator's contributions to the interaction and that "other indicators are needed to reflect the child's contributions when the concerns are diagnostic or research related, and there are times when more complex coding systems are relevant for capturing the complex interactional effects" *(page 69)*.

For the purposes of the current volume, the MLE Rating Scale is useful for assessors to monitor their own interventions in test-mediate-retest DAs. It may also be used in the counselling of parents and carers, and the evaluation of the extent of mediation in their interactions, in a manner similar to that of Parent-Child Interaction Therapy.

A simplified record of the presence or absence of mediational inputs by examiners was used by Hasson (2011). The behaviours recorded were derived from those described by Haywood (1993) as the 'Unique Character of Teacher-Mediated Interactions'. Six behaviours were identified, as previously described in Chapter 2. Speech and language therapy sessions were videotaped, and each instance of the target behaviour was counted. A simple count such as this is useful as a reminder to assessors to include essential mediations in their assessments.

The presence or absence of mediational behaviours in assessors was subsequently slightly extended in a pilot project carried out by the author, which looked at the reliability of the implementation of a DA by SLTs new to the process (unpublished data). Fifteen-minute segments of video were sampled, which were thought to be representative of the sessions and which were long enough to allow the SLT and the child to become accustomed to the procedure, as well as to contain easier and more challenging items.

Scoring of the presence of mediation made use of a specially constructed scoresheet, based on the instructions that SLTs were given about implementing mediated intervention. The mediational behaviours were ones that SLTs might have been expected to include for each of the items and at any level of the prompt hierarchy. Four components of MLE and eight additional specific behaviours were identified and used to construct a scale for rating the presence or absence of the mediational behaviours.

For example, rating of an MLE item was presented as follows:

Mediation of transcendence – linking the activity to other contexts in which the skill can be used, "promotion of cognitive bridges between the task or activity and related but not currently present experiences of the child; these may refer to the past or may anticipate the future".

For example: Reference to tasks in the past or future:

Elaborated hypothetical, inferential or cause and effect thinking.

PRESENT /ABSENT

Rating of an additional behaviour was presented as follows:

Ask questions – *i.e. elicit rather than give answers.*
Asking the child what to do rather than telling him.

PRESENT /ABSENT

The videos were marked according to observation of the presence of the 12 aspects at any one time in the brief segment of video, and results were summarised on a scoresheet which appears in Appendix B08 and may be useful as a template for monitoring an assessor's use of mediation.

In the pilot study, independent ratings of mediational behaviours using this scale were found to be reliable. All of the SLTS used three of the types of mediational behaviours (Intentionality, Meaning and Applying Rules), but in general, SLTs need to attend to the implementation of intervention that contains the remaining nine mediational behaviours.

Ratings of modifiability

The 'other indicators' referred to by Lidz gave rise to the development of the Response to Mediation Scale (RtM Lidz 2003). This scale is focused on the child or recipient of mediational intervention and is completed after observation of a mediated intervention session.

Each of 11 behaviours of the learner, labelled A to K, is rated on a five-point scale, consisting of a description of responses for the behaviour. The full scale is included in Appendix B09. Examples of the descriptors are as follows:

A. Self-regulation of attention

1   Unable to maintain attention to task
2   Fleeting attention to task even with input from adult
3   Maintains with significant input from adult
4   Maintains with occasional input from adult
5   Maintains with no input from adult
Does not apply

G. Responsiveness to initiations of mediator

1   Resistant to mediator's initiatives
2   Passive noncompliant
3   Passive minimally responsive

4   Consistently responsive

5   Enthusiastic and responsive

Does not apply

The RtM scale is extremely useful for capturing the characteristics of the child in the intervention session and provides useful information for the planning of intervention. As children with language disorders do not necessarily have generalised cognitive difficulties, several of the sections may be excluded and only the ones felt to be most relevant included.

A similar scale developed by Peña, and described in Peña, Resendiz and Gillam (2007), is the Mediated Learning Observation (MLO) scale. Previous research indicated that clinicians' ratings of a child's modifiability were good predictors of language disorder. The MLO scale consists of 12 behavioural items, which are thought to influence the way that children learn. Each behaviour is scored from 1 to 5, according to descriptors, where 1 is mastery and 5 indicates a high level of need in the given area (see Appendix B10). The behaviours are arranged into four categories:

1   Internal social-emotional (affect)

- anxiety

- motivation

- non-verbal persistence

2   Cognitive arousal (ability to resist distraction)

- task orientation

- metacognition

- non-verbal self-reward

3   Cognitive elaboration (thinking)

- problem solving

- verbal mediation

- flexibility

4   External social-emotional (behaviour)

- responsiveness to feedback

- attention

- compliance

Peña *et al.* were able to demonstrate that children with and without DLD performed differently on the scale, particularly in the areas of cognitive arousal and elaboration. Clinicians were able to accurately categorise children into typical or language disordered on the basis of a combination of two measures of modifiability, namely metacognition (indicated by child awareness of performance and of errors) and flexibility (indicated by use of change in strategy). Similarly, some of the measures on the rating scale correlated highly with the gains made on the pre- and post-narrative tests.

For clinical purposes, the MLO scale can be used alongside the mediational intervention session(s) of a DA to add diagnostic information, or to inform the clinician about the additional factors affecting the child's learning. This adds to prognostic or predictive value of the assessment, as well as indicating targets for intervention.

When mediational interventions are used as part of the test-train-retest DA, the scoring of the DA should contain measures of the impact of training on general cognitive performance as well as gains in language. Followers of Feuerstein and users of his assessment instruments, for example Tzuriel *et al.* (1999), use achievement tests along with tests of task-intrinsic motivation and metacognitive activity to evaluate the effects of a mediational intervention programme.

Summary

In summary, scoring may be based on

quantitative data

rating scales

observational or qualitative data

Quantitative data may be a count of

criteria reached – i.e. curriculum based or the items on a static test;

number of prompts introduced to the child to enable task completion;

levels of prompts reached; and

number of attempts made by the child before the task is solved.

Rating scales may be used to

evaluate the mediational input by the assessor;

rate examiner effort; and

identify significant factors in the child's response to the intervention.

Observational or qualitative data would relate to

the child's utterances or responses to the task or the facilitations (or mediations);

additional knowledge, such as metacognitive awareness;

use of problem-solving strategies; and

specific content or linguistic difficulties.

Furthermore, scoring may be carried out at the following stages:

at static pre-test;

during the training phase of a test-train-retest;

during a graded prompting task;

at post-test; and

pre-post-test scores may be compared to calculate gain.

Improvement from item to item within the training may be quantified to evaluate ongoing learning and transfer.

We will see how some of these are used in the DASS in the next chapter.

References

Carlson, J.S., and Wiedl, K.H. (1978) 'Use of testing-the-limits procedures in the assessment of intellectual capabilities in children with learning difficulties', *American Journal of Mental Deficiency*, 82(6), pp. 559–564.

Embretson, S.E. (1987) 'Improving the measurement of spatial aptitude by dynamic testing', *Intelligence*, 11(4), pp. 333–358.

Feuerstein, R., Feuerstein, R.S., Falik, L.H. and Rand, Y. (2002) *The dynamic assessment of cognitive modifiability: The learning propensity assessment device: Theory, instruments and techniques*, ICELP Press, Jerusalem.

Guthke, J., Beckmann, J.F., and Dobat, H. (1997) 'Dynamic testing problems, uses, trends and evidence of validity', *Educational and Child Psychology*, 14(4), pp. 17–32.

Hasson, N. (2011). *Dynamic assessment and informed intervention for children with language impairment.* (Unpublished Doctoral thesis) City University London. Online, http://openaccess.city. ac.uk/1119/

Hasson, N., Nash, L., Cubie, B., Kessie, A. and Marshall, C. (2014) *Dynamic assessment of morphological analysis: A UK based study.* Poster presented to RCSLT Conference, University of Leeds.

Haywood, H.C. (1993) 'A mediational teaching style', *International Journal of Cognitive Education and Mediated Learning*, 3(1), pp. 27–38.

Larsen, J.A., and Nippold, M.A. (2007) 'Morphological analysis in school-age children: Dynamic assessment of a word learning strategy', *Language, Speech, and Hearing Services in Schools*, 38(3), pp. 201–212.

Lidz, C.S. (1991) *Practitioner's guide to dynamic assessment*, The Guilford Press, New York.

Lidz, C.S. (2003) *Early childhood assessment*, Wiley, Hoboken, NJ.

Peña, E.D., Resendiz, M. and Gillam, R.B. (2007) 'The role of clinical judgements of modifiability in the diagnosis of language impairment', *International Journal of Speech-Language Pathology*, 9(4), pp. 332–345.

Ram, G., Marinellie, S.A., Benigno, J. and McCarthy, J. (2013) 'Morphological analysis in context versus isolation: Use of a dynamic assessment task with school-age children', *Language, Speech, and Hearing Services in Schools*, 44, pp. 32–47.

Resing, W.C.M. (1997) 'Learning potential assessment: The alternative for measuring intelligence?', *Educational and Child Psychology*, 14, pp. 68–82.

Resing, W.C.M., De Jong, F.M., Bosma, T. and Tunteler, E. (2009) 'Learning during dynamic testing: Variability in strategy use by indigenous and ethnic minority children', *Journal of Cognitive Education and Psychology*, 8(1), pp. 22–37.

Swanson, H.L., and Lussier, C.M. (2001) 'A selective synthesis of the experimental literature on dynamic assessment', *Review of Educational Research*, 71(2), pp. 321–349.

Tzuriel, D., Kaniel, S., Kanner, E. and Haywood, H.C. (1999) 'Effects of the "Bright Start" program in kindergarten on transfer and academic achievement', *Early Childhood Research Quarterly*, 14(1), pp. 111–141.

Chapter 5
The DASS

Aim of the DASS research

Materials

    The test items

    Structure of the DA

    Procedure

The mediational prompt structure

Scoring

Trials of the DASS

In this chapter, we will take a close look at a DA designed for the assessment of the grammatical sentence skills of school-age children with language impairments: the DASS (Hasson 2011; Hasson, Dodd and Botting 2012). The method and materials exemplify many of the principles that have been presented in the foregoing chapters and illustrate the choices and decisions that were made in the construction of the instrument. The findings of the trials of the DASS are also reported. All of the materials for administration of the DASS are available in Appendix A.

Aim of the DASS research

The aim of the research was to formulate a procedure for DA of language that yielded useful information for planning intervention for children with language disorders. The test was intended to be statistically valid and reliable, and the procedure needed to be replicable and teachable so that it could be adopted by practising SLTs in the field. Furthermore, for it to be clinically useful, the administration time and scoring simplicity needed to be controlled.

The DASS was not intended to be diagnostic in the sense that it differentiates children with language disorders from typically developing children, but rather it was intended to add more detail and clinically useful information to the profiles of children already identified as having disordered language.

The target population for the test is children aged approximately eight to ten years, although there is some flexibility around the ages because there is no need to match to the criteria of a normative population. For this reason, the test may be useful for slightly older or younger children, depending on the severity of their language impairments. The procedure is also useful for children with language disorders accompanied by other conditions such as ADHD and mild learning difficulties.

Materials

The task is a sentence anagram, based on the 'Sentence Assembly' subtest of the CELF-3 (UK) (Semel, Wiig and Secord 1987). The words are presented visually, printed on a single card in random order. The child is required to formulate two possible sentences from the given words. It was chosen for the present test because it enables the assessor to look at a number of underlying component skills and processes through a careful task analysis, as discussed in Chapter 3.

For example, we would present the task without instructions to see whether the child is able to determine that the words as presented do not make sense and that he may need to rearrange them. Verbalising this would indicate whether the child has a grasp of metalinguistic concepts such as 'words', 'sentences', 'making sense' and 'the right order'. We would also record whether he is able to express these ideas, knows the vocabulary and is able to formulate the meanings appropriately. At this point, we might also note the child's ability to read the words correctly, as although the DA is not a test of reading, we do need to know whether he may have done poorly on standardised tests because of poor reading and whether he is able to use the written words to aid memory during the sentence arrangement task.

The task reduces the demand on short-term memory by having the words written and in view throughout the task. There is still, however, a demand for working memory, as the child has to hold the sequence of words in mind as he formulates the sentence. Presenting the words on separate cards that could be moved around is an alternative method that would eliminate the need for working memory, but as it has been shown to be a key skill in linguistic formulation, and one that has been shown to be poor in children with language disorders (Gathercole and Baddeley 1993), the need for working memory in the task was retained. The assessor can observe the child's performance in this area and any strategies that the child uses to manage the memory demand of the task.

Two parallel versions of the materials for the DA are available, to enable assessors to repeat the test at different times. This may be used to monitor progress. Each version contains the identical sentence constructions, with different vocabulary items and names inserted into the sentences. All of the vocabulary used is everyday vocabulary of nouns and verbs thought to be well within the experience of children of primary age. The procedure, however, also allows the assessor to explain any unknown vocabulary to participants.

The grammatical structure of the possible sentences in the DASS is tightly controlled and sequenced so that different linguistic constructions are required in each item. They are presented in order of increasing difficulty, and/or increasing sentence length or number of items in the sentence, for each grammatical structure. This structure enables the assessor to see if the child is able to retain what he has learnt and transfer strategies from one item to the next, as the test progresses.

As an example, item 3 contains reversible content in a Subject-Verb (SVcSV) construction:

Mum is eating and Dad is drinking.

Item 4 then repeats the reversible content to assess whether the strategy has been learnt and retained for use in the next item, but also increases the length of the sentence to Subject-Verb-Object (SVOcSVO):

Mum is driving the car and Dad is riding the bike.

The nature of the child's attempts will indicate whether he knows how to structure the sentence and reverse the content and whether he is confused by the longer SVO clause structure. It also affords opportunity to observe whether the child is aware of the semantic constraints that *riding* is associated with a bike and *driving* with a car.

By requiring two different sentences to be made, the task taps directly into the individual's ability to manipulate linguistic elements to encode different grammatical relationships. For example, the sentence "*The boy is washing my car*" and the question "*Is the boy washing my car?*" can be formulated from the same set of words, within the rules of grammar which the child must know. Individuals frequently recognise one sentence immediately or easily, but the challenge of the second sentence is to show cognitive flexibility and not get stuck on the first sentence. In addition, the individual needs to employ linguistic knowledge more explicitly and actively problem solve to work out a second sentence. This is where opportunities to mediate cognitive strategies, reinforce linguistic rules and observe the ability of the individual to learn from the input become important.

Finally, the specific linguistic structures that were tested by the developed materials were selected in part to represent structures known to be impaired in the language of children with language disorders, for example, auxiliary verb reversal, copula verbs and pronouns. The order of presentation of sentence items takes account of grammatical complexity and sequence of age of acquisition. This is in order to facilitate training through the presentation and practice of the test items themselves. The test also begins with simpler examples in order to give children confidence and to ease the fear of failure and reluctance to participate that affects their performance on assessment tasks.

The grammatical structures of each utterance are shown in Appendix A04.

The test items

The items used in the A and B versions of the test and the materials for presentation can be found in Appendix A.

Structure of the DA

The DASS is basically constructed as a graduated prompting procedure. There is no static pre- or post-test, although many children may in the past have completed the Sentence Assembly subtest of the CELF.

The test/training procedure is carried out in one session, or possibly two if the child has not completed the items because of the lengthy training time being required, or because of fatigue. All 12 items are presented, as they cover a range of grammatical structures that are in themselves a source of information about the child's linguistic knowledge. The items must be presented in the given sequence because of the increasing level of grammatical complexity of the items.

The items are first presented to the child for him to solve independently, and cues are provided only when required to help the child solve the problem item. There are five levels of help available, defined by the general type of information and nature of assistance. The actual cues are not prescribed or scripted, but may be expressed, and are mediated, in a flexible and individualised way, depending on the needs of the child and his responses during the test.

The cues are graded from general metacognitive direction, or no specific prompt (level 1), to strategy-based suggestions (levels 2–3), breaking down the task into components and using specific feedback (level 4) and finally to item-specific feedback and instruction (level 5). The prompt sheet that may be used during the DA can be found in Appendix A05.

1 Metacognitive direction
2 Drawing on previous knowledge
3 Finding strategies
  Problem solving
4 Breaking down the task
  Using specific feedback
5 Learning from feedback and instruction

Procedure

At the start, the child is asked, "Do you know what you have to do?" and "Can you tell me what you have to do?" The response can be used to evaluate metacognitive awareness of task requirements.

The child should be allowed time to respond to each item without prompting from the assessor. Incomplete attempts are supported with "Yes, go on". When the child indicates that he is in difficulty, the prompts are introduced sequentially.

Wording of the prompts is variable and mediational in nature, allowing children to find their own solutions as far as possible and to make judgements or justify their attempts.

When the items are complete, children are asked reflective questions, such as "How did you know how to do that?" "Was it easy or hard?" "What was hard?" or "What made that one easy?" These responses are only used to evaluate metacognitive awareness.

The level of prompting that has been reached can be scored for each item as the test progresses using the scoresheets (see Appendix A06 and A07).The scoresheet is completed with a tick in the appropriate column. If children are curious about the scoring, the sheet can be shared with them, and the assessor explains that where they have been given a tick in the first column, they have completed the item 'all by themselves', whereas other items were difficult and "I needed to help you a bit". There are no instances where there is no tick, where the item has not been solved, and so no record of failure.

The mediational prompt structure

The style of interaction adopted by the examiner should be mediational, as recommended by Feuerstein and described by Lidz (1991), as presented in Chapter 2.

The session should incorporate essential mediational components in that there should be clear transmission of intentionality and meaning to the child, mediation of competence (lots of praise and encouragement) and task regulation (reducing guessing and impulsiveness) throughout, as well as transcendence or bridging of the skills to other applications. Mediation of any component during the training procedure is allowed but should not detract from the essential sequence of the cues, or distract the child or examiner from the task.

Lidz (2003 p. 121) noted that other MLE components are assumed to automatically be included by an examiner in a mediational intervention session. Mediation of metacognitive strategies such as planning, self-regulation and checking, that are domain general and not specific to the task at hand, may be included and have been reported to facilitate generalisation.

In addition, some children may be asked questions relating to linguistic structures in order to identify metalinguistic knowledge that could inform intervention, or for the assessor to gain insights into the problem solving and grammatical knowledge of the child. For example, children might be asked "Which is the person or 'doing word' in this sentence?" Or, "What is meant by the 's'" (possessive apostrophe) in one item, to which some children in the author's experience replied that it signified a plural.

We will now take a look at the prompts in more detail.

1   The score of 1 is given when the item is completed spontaneously; in other words, the child arranges the words into a grammatical sentence without any assistance from the examiner.

The cue "*Do you know what you have to do?*" is an introduction to the task, adds insights into whether the child is aware of the problem (that the words don't make sense in the given order) and assesses his ability to identify and explain the task, including his vocabulary and sentence structure. This is qualitative information only. *The child does not have to answer the question in order to score the point;* he need only produce a correct sentence. Note that once the child has done one or two items, the introduction will be redundant, and the assessor will only need to present the next card.

2   Level 2 relates to general, non-specific, non-linguistic cues. When the child does not respond spontaneously, he may need to be prompted to look at the words, confirm that he is able to read them and think about whether he may have done a similar task before. Children with attention difficulties may be refocused to the task at hand, and children with learning difficulties might not have grasped what is required of them. At this point, the examiner may need to help the child read some of the words or explain any unfamiliar vocabulary, which does, on occasion, enable the child to then complete the item. Clearly, this is very informative for future management.

3   The third level is the point at which concrete help is given to the child in the form of strategies and problem-solving methods. What is important is that these are *transferable* strategies and are not related to the particular item presented. If the child learns to follow a *process* of reasoning or problem solving, his own thinking is modified for the future, which is the ultimate goal of mediational intervention. So at this stage, it is important to teach strategic planning, checking and use of rules.

Questions that might be used are as follows:

- *Which one can you start with?* Mediating systematic planning rather than trial and error or guessing. This is also an opportunity to teach about grammar – that sentences start with the Subject, a person, which is often enough for this to be a useful place to start looking for the structure, or that a question might start with '*Is*'.

- *Can you make little groups of words?* Again, mediation is used to help the child break down the task, link meaningful units together to reduce the overall load and manipulate the phrases in a sentence. At this level, this is suggested as a strategy; if the child needs help to carry out the process, it will be a level 4 or 5 prompt. Try not to provide the extra help too early, but allow the child to use the information or cues he has to solve the task himself.

- *Can you make a different kind of sentence? A question?* As noted earlier, it is preferable to avoid telling the child to make a question, but the concept of 'a different kind of sentence' may be too abstract. It is still a strategy related to the anagram task, but not to the individual item, as it recurs in later items, and the retention of question formation as a strategy signals the learning of problem solving.

- *Can you swap the words around?* A concrete strategy is suggested without actually demonstrating how the items would appear.

- A final strategy for making a second sentence with the same words might be to rearrange structures already formed for the first sentence. So, again, specific to the anagram task but not to any particular item:

    "What did you say before?" Or, "Last time you said . . ."

This reinforces the child's active role in the problem solving and demonstrates to him that his own contribution is valuable.

Also in Level 3 are cues directing the child to the rules of the task that they might have overlooked. Adherence to the rules of a task is an important strategy, and mediation of rule-governed behaviour facilitates learning and problem solving in a wide range of situations. Checking one's own responses is also essential to effective performance.

- *Have you used all the words?*

- *What have you left out?*

- *Have you used any of the words more than once?*

- *Does it make sense?*

4   At level 4, item-specific prompts are given. The task can be broken down for the child or specific feedback given. At this stage. the assessor is still asking questions to lead the child to discover the answer for himself, but the guidance is more specific and uses the item content. The process of solving the particular item is mediated to the child; it is systematic, sequenced and rule governed, and the child needs to discover the system, the sequence and the rules.

   At this stage, the child is probably making attempts to solve the item and form sentences, so specific feedback can be given – for example, *"Do you have the word 'to?'" "No you don't, that's right, so it can't be 'Give to. . .' it must be 'Give. . .?' 'Give Mummy' "*.

Examples of questions are as follows:

- *Which one can you start with?* Mediating the strategy of systematic planning. Note that the question is now followed up with the specific item 'John' rather than "Start with the person". It is accompanied by pointing to the target word. Similarly, "*Which one can you start with to make a question?*" If needed, the follow-up prompt would be '*Start with X'*

- *What comes next?*

- *What is this word? What does it go with?* So perhaps "*Let's keep 'brush your teeth' together and 'go to bed'. Now think about which one comes first?*"

- *Does that make sense?* This is used when the answer given is both correct and incorrect to facilitate reflection as well as judgement and correction. It may be used when the sentence is semantically inappropriate e.g. "*Does the window break if you cry?*" It is always important that the child knows why the sentence is wrong so that he can correct the error, or try again, and he needs to learn to spot errors for himself. Therefore, if the sentence is correct, he is also asked to justify it, "*How do you know it's right?*"

- *You've left this one out. Where does it go?*

- *Repeat part of the answer already used.* Particularly in longer sentences, the examiner might present part of the sentence already constructed by the child, for completion. "*The boy is going to . . . ?*" This breaks down the task into smaller components and enables the use of an elimination strategy in which the child can acknowledge the words already used and see what words remain.

- *Giving part of the answer.* This cue is similar to the previous one and presents the task as a sentence completion task. A trial of this type of facilitation informs plans for future intervention.

5 The level 5 cue is the highest level of prompting, or the one in which the most intensive support is provided. The sentence is scaffolded word by word, and requests for imitation may be made. The whole sentence may need to be provided, or a cloze task may be presented that requires a word to be added. Specific feedback is provided in instances where the child is not able to provide the responses himself. Although the input is item specific, the examiner may still use the mediational tool of 'bridging' – i.e. relating the learning to another instance in which the same learning might apply. So, for example, the assessor might say, "*Is the girl reading a book? That's a question about what someone is doing isn't it? So your Mum might say, 'Johnny, are you doing your homework? Or you say, 'Is Dad watching TV?' then you will know where everyone is and what they are doing. Why might we want to know that? Maybe you can't see where Dad is, and you need to ask Mum*".

Finally, when the prompting is complete and the answers have been produced, children are asked to reflect on the process.

Examples of questions are as follows:

- *Is that the right answer? Why was it not OK?*
- *Can you tell me how you did that?*
- *How did you know how to do that?*
- *Was it easy or hard? Why?*

When a correct solution is presented, the examiner prompts the child for a reflective response, primarily a judgement of grammaticality and sense, as well as an evaluation by the child of the strategies he used and the level of difficulty he experienced. This procedure was also described by Gutierrez-Clellen and Peña (2001) as a variation on the 'Testing the Limits' procedure, and it was found to enable children to demonstrate their knowledge better and the examiner to understand the child's thinking and approach to problem solving better. Reflection is intended to facilitate improved generalisation as recommended by Peña, Resendiz and Gillam (2007 p. 335) and to provide opportunity for further metacognitive mediation, which promotes transfer of gains (Keane 1987). Mediated prompting after level 5 of the procedure is not scored or regarded as part of the graduated prompt structure, but it is an essential part of the mediational intervention.

Scoring

The number of cues presented is recorded on the scoresheet (see Appendix A06) as the procedure is carried out. The number of each type of cue can be totalled immediately after completion of the assessment session by a count of the number of ticks in each column.

As there are two responses required for each item, one for each sentence formed from the words, scoring is based on a total of 24 responses. Each of the 24 items is scored between 1 and 5, therefore there is a total score, with a minimum of 24 and a maximum of 120.

In addition, there is a tally of the number of each level of cue required: how many ones, twos, etc. were required. This gives information about the learning needs of the individual throughout the whole procedure, elucidating whether he requires mostly strategy training or item-specific application of knowledge.

Qualitative measures are also used to inform future intervention:

i)   Identification of grammatical structures which caused the child the greatest difficulty.

ii) The effect of the amount of content (sentence length) and nature of semantic content on the child's construction of linguistic structures.

iii) The child's ability to transfer, or generalise, learning or strategies – i.e. item-to-item transfer – as well as which items benefited from transfer effects.

iv) The child's metalinguistic knowledge, ability to label, explain and manipulate linguistic concepts.

v) The child's metacognitive ability – i.e. awareness of the processes and strategies that are used to solve the given task.

Trials of the DASS

In the original trial of the DASS (Hasson, Dodd and Botting 2012), the cohort consisted of 24 children, aged between 8.2 and 10.9. All were referred by SLTs working with the children in language resource bases and a special school for children with communication disorders, and all had language disorders identified as the primary disorder, with children scoring < 1 standard deviation (SD) below the mean for age on a standardised language test. They were required to have English as a first language, but no learning difficulties, (IQ > 70), hearing impairments or attention deficit disorders.

The nature of the study required that the investigator carry out all the DA testing. In order to control for experimenter bias, an independent assessor videotaped and scored the assessments.

Scores from the CELF-3(UK) at the start of the study were compared to DASS scores to establish concurrent validity of the procedure. At the conclusion of the study, SLTs treating the participants in the study were asked via a questionnaire whether they found the information arising out of the DA useful.

The results of the study showed that all of the children scored poorly on the CELF-3(UK) (Semel, Wiig and Secord 1987), with standard scores of 20 out of the 24 children at least 2.5 SD below the mean for age, scoring below the first percentile.

In contrast, DASS scores of the whole cohort were widely distributed, with a mean score of 61.83 and standard deviation of 20.72. Although the distribution was skewed to the lower end, this was predictable given the language-impaired nature of the sample. No limiting floor or ceiling effects were found. A significant correlation was found between participants' scores on the DASS and total raw scores on the CELF-3 (UK) ($rs = -0.481$, $p = 0.017$). The correlation is in a negative direction, as greater ability on the CELF obtains a higher score, while stronger performance on the DASS is shown by need for fewer prompt cues and hence a lower score. The correlation observed is moderate as would be expected, as only part of the DASS score is related to language knowledge, which is assessed by the CELF.

Inter-rater reliability of scoring revealed a significant correlation between the total scores for each participant ($n = 6$) for each rater ($rs = 0.886$, $p = 0.019$).

The study concluded that the aim to create a reliable and valid DA of sentence-level language had been achieved. In addition, the high correlation between the scoring of the experimenter and an independent rater with minimal training, as well as the positive responses obtained from SLTs, suggested that the procedure would be replicable and useful to practising SLTs.

In a subsequent trial, 10 volunteer practicing speech and language therapists trialled the procedure on 17 children from their own caseloads. All SLTs were trained in the DASS procedure by the experimenter in small group sessions lasting approximately 90 minutes and including video examples. Participating SLTs were provided with all of the materials for the procedure as well as a three-page handout that explained the dynamic and mediational aspects of the assessments and gave guidelines for mediation. Specific practice in mediational techniques was not given, although the training video was accompanied by commentary. Participating SLTs were also reassured that any queries about test administration and scoring would be answered by email, and a small number of SLTs took up this opportunity to clarify requirements.

SLTs were asked to recruit a minimum of two clients from their own caseloads for the study. Criteria for inclusion of the children were as follows:

1   Children with previously identified language impairments, currently attending SLT for language disorder. Children with language disorders associated with other disorders were not excluded.
2   Age range approximately eight to ten years, although SLTs were invited to try the procedure on a wider age range if they thought the procedure might be applicable to the child.
3   Consent to record the child and make de-identified data available to the researcher.

A total of 17 videos with completed scoresheets were received. The children about whom feedback was received from the SLTs (n = 16) ranged in age from 7.11 to 11.2, with one additional sample of a child aged 15.3. Nine children were identified as language impaired, two as language impaired with additional attention difficulties, one as language impaired with autistic spectrum disorder (ASD) and one as language impaired with additional learning difficulties. A further child was diagnosed as ASD and one with learning difficulty, without language impairment being identified. One participant recruited from a SLT's caseload was undiagnosed at the time of the study and was subsequently discharged from the service.

The researcher scored the test from the videos, blind to the original scoring, and subsequently compared results with the scores of the SLT.

The researcher also re-watched a 15-minute segment of the first video from each SLT. Scoring of the mediation made use of a specially constructed scoresheet for the rating of the presence or absence of the mediational behaviours. The researcher and an independent scorer with some experience in DA rated the videos independently, and the scores were correlated for a measure of rater reliability. Rating of the criteria by the experimenter and the independent rater correlated highly, $r_s = 0.890$, $p < 0.01$.

The study showed that despite reporting uncertainty in the scoring of the test, the SLTs in the study were highly reliable in their quantitative scoring of the levels of prompting used in the DASS. This again confirmed that the hierarchy of cues is transparent, while still allowing for some individual flexibility in the wording of questions and prompts to support the individual children.

However, the SLTs varied considerably in their technique of administration of the test, which was captured by the rating of the presence of mediational behaviours. The use of mediation to establish the needs of individuals for support was considered important by the author of the test because it contributes to the depth of information about the individual child that can be extracted from the procedure. It was felt that, overall, while the prompting by SLTs was mediational in nature, the SLTs missed some opportunities to probe the metacognitive awareness of the children. Four of the 10 SLTs, none of whom had prior experience in administering DAs, demonstrated 9 or more of the 12 components of a mediational intervention and showed that they grasped the mediational principles well. Five could have benefited from more instruction or explicit training in mediation and one struggled to administer the task with any degree of fidelity.

Therapists fed back that they felt unsure about some aspects of the test administration and scoring procedures and would clearly have benefited from more instruction. Some slight modifications to the test items themselves were also recommended. The study reflected that the procedure, like all assessments, was not suitable for all children. The inclusion of children for whom the test was not applicable was a limitation of the project, but contributed information useful for future modifications of the procedure.

Nevertheless, clinicians responded to the feedback questionnaire positively, elaborating in many cases on how they found the additional data to be useful.

Conclusion

This study contributed to the conception and planning of the current text, which explores the theory and practice of DA in greater detail before presenting a detailed manual for administration of the DASS. This chapter should be read in conjunction with the materials presented in Appendix A, which are reproducible for the use of professionals employing the DA in their clinical work.

References

Gathercole, S.E., and Baddeley, A.D. (1993) *Working memory and language*, Psychology Press, Hove.

Gutierrez-Clellen, V.F., and Peña, E. (2001) 'Dynamic assessment of diverse children: A tutorial', *Language, Speech, and Hearing Services in Schools*, 32(4), pp. 212–224.

Hasson, N. (2011). *Dynamic assessment and informed intervention for children with language impairment.* (Unpublished Doctoral thesis) City University London. Online, http://openaccess.city.ac.uk/1119/

Hasson, N., Dodd, B. and Botting, N. (2012) 'Dynamic Assessment of Sentence Structure (DASS): Design and evaluation of a novel procedure for assessment of syntax in children with language impairments', *International Journal of Language and Communication Disorders*, 47(3), pp. 285–299.

Keane, K.J. (1987) 'Assessing deaf children', Lidz, C.S. (ed) *Dynamic assessment: An interactional approach to evaluating learning potential*, Guilford Press, New York.

Lidz, C.S. (1991) *Practitioner's guide to dynamic assessment*, The Guilford Press, New York.

Lidz, C.S. (2003) *Early childhood assessment*, Wiley, Hoboken, NJ.

Peña, E.D., Resendiz, M. and Gillam, R.B. (2007) 'The role of clinical judgements of modifiability in the diagnosis of language impairment', *International Journal of Speech-Language Pathology*, 9(4), pp. 332–345.

Semel, E., Wiig, E.H. and Secord, W. (1987) *Clinical evaluation of language fundamentals*, 3rd edn, The Psychological Corporation, London.

Chapter 6
Applications to intervention

Interpretation of DA of language

Case examples

Reporting of a DA

Interpreting the responses made during a DA has been mentioned several times in the previous chapters. The information elicited from a DA is considerably more detailed and complex than a numerical score that relates to a normative population.

Primarily, a DA aims to evaluate 'potential to learn'. To evaluate this, we need to interpret the responsiveness to intervention, or improvement through the short period of learning incorporated in the DA, which determines immediate potential for change in individuals. In a qualitative way, responses to the mediation and different facilitative cues inform the practitioner about the likely response of the individual to different intervention programmes, and can enable prognosis for improvement to be established.

Further, a DA can help to identify what cognitive processes are weak, and can benefit from intervention, and which are stable and used to support weak(er) language skills.

According to Haywood and Lidz (2007), an assessment that clarifies the problem and generates hypotheses appropriately leads in a logical way to good intervention.

Interpretation of DA of language

We have seen that the assessment of aspects of language is based not on the product but on the process. Linguistic tasks are frequently complex, requiring efficient processing of incoming language and information, access to a knowledge base and memory functions, as well as formulation and expression of a response. There may be limitations in the input phase, the elaboration or the output (Feuerstein *et al.* 2002). We do not need a DA to identify the gaps or errors in a child's language output, but we can benefit from a better understanding of where the breakdown lies and *how* the individual is attempting to complete the task.

Looking at the performance of children on the DASS, for example, we can see that a considerable amount of difficulty that particularly affects the grammatical elements identified in the table would suggest a specifically linguistic basis to the child's impairment. For example, the child might consistently omit the auxiliary verb in his sentences and produce "*the man painting the wall*"*. He may offer this as a complete sentence to the assessor and fail to self-correct on the basis of checking that he has used all the words.

Implicit, and sometimes explicit, in the DASS task is the request for children to make judgements of grammaticality, which is known to be difficult for children with language disorders (Gopnik and Crago, 1991; Wulfeck and Bates 1995, cited by Leonard 1998). Children are asked to judge whether the sentences are correct. The examiner frequently facilitates this judgement task by repeating the sentence back to the child so that he can make judgements based on a fluent auditory model. This helps to reduce the processing load and enables some children to demonstrate their syntactic knowledge.

Alternatively, a child who is more obviously affected by the number of items, or semantic constraints on sentences, or who fails to transfer learning from one item to the next, may be seen to have more domain general processing problems, or there may be signs of limitations on working memory capacity (Marton and Schwartz 2003). Strategies to manage these should then be addressed in therapy.

Case examples

Peña and Gillam (2000) explicitly linked DAs to recommendations for intervention in a series of three cases. The reader is referred to the chapter for the full explanation of the DA process and interpretation of the findings.

In the course of the author's professional SLT career, and during the research into the DASS, numerous interesting cases emerged. The principles of test interpretation leading to planning might best be presented via the following examples.

Child O: Aged five, attending a language resource
O participated in a DA of vocabulary. He was unable to use the strategy of eliminating pictures that he knew in order to identify an unknown label. As a result, his attempts were entirely trial and error. Not only was there reduced vocabulary but also cognitive limitations that restricted his learning of new words.

Child P: Aged nine

The following is an excerpt from the findings of the DASS:

> P was able to arrange most of the sentences independently and seemed to find the structured task easier than having to formulate expressive language spontaneously. His expressive language is characterised by long and rambling constructions and a lack of precision in getting his meaning across. There is a lack of detail and accuracy, resulting in confusion of some structures e.g. articles and pronouns.
>
> P attempted to impose order on his responses and explain or justify what he had produced; however, these explanations were imprecise, and P did not seem to have the vocabulary and concepts to explain himself. His metalinguistic knowledge is implicit; he indicated that he was aware of the manipulations of words to form sentences, but was unable to express them clearly. There is a need for P to increase his metalinguistic vocabulary alongside syntactic expression to reason linguistically and to develop higher-level language structures. P has a good semantic understanding and appreciates absurdity and humour, although the structural details are not grasped; for example, he cannot identify that a single word has two meanings.
>
> In the first CELF-3 test, P's expressive language score was higher than his receptive language, and although this may be an artefact of testing, P's attention to detail and careful gathering of information may be impaired so that he does not fully process incoming language. He has difficulty following instructions and checking that he has planned his responses carefully. His teacher identified several functional difficulties related to attending to and processing verbal information, instructions and rules.
>
> In summary, it would appear that P's typical performance does not reflect the extent of his knowledge. He would benefit from improvement of his cognitive functioning – increasing awareness and control over behaviours such as careful gathering of information; attention to detail, checking, selecting and planning his responses; and reflecting on his performance. He demonstrated responsiveness and understanding of some of these concepts during the DA. These generalisable skills may enable him to perform better in language tasks and in class.

Child L: Aged six

During a DA, L was found to have some conceptual difficulties. He struggled to recognise the elements in pictures and to interpret them. He confused *hot* and *cold*, and was unable to relate the labels to winter/summer, or to the wearing of a coat.

It was recommended that intervention make use of concrete examples to add meaning to everyday concepts and that concepts be addressed on a single or two-word level before the morphological and syntactic elements of language were tackled.

Child E: Aged eight
Observations of E's language included

- stable use of the SVO structure;

- lack of awareness that 'isn't' has the same function as 'is';

- recognition of plural '-s', but inability to explain the concept;

- inability to recognize possessive 's';

- difficulty arranging elements of a sentence using 'after' — confused temporal sequence;

- inclined to attempt grammatically correct but semantically illogical sentences;

- cannot identify the action (or 'doing word') in a sentence; and

- sometimes uncertain of judgement of grammaticality.

Summary after DA:

- E has structural regularity in her expressive language and can formulate basic sentences reliably. She still has considerable difficulty with grammatical morphemes and formulating more varied sentence structures accurately; this is exacerbated by uncertainty in making judgements of correctness.

- She demonstrates metalinguistic awareness and knowledge, and attempts to use strategic problem solving spontaneously.

- E has good interpersonal communication skills and a willingness to engage and to learn.

- E may require ongoing SLT intervention to address both receptive and expressive language difficulties, focusing on structural features of language and morphology, but her inclination to try to transfer and generalise what she has learnt may facilitate learning of systematic rule-governed aspects.

- Intervention might, therefore, make use of explicit rule teaching and application.

- As E is uncertain about her own judgements of correct grammar; it may be useful to carry out activities requiring judgement as well as justification for her choices based on rules she has learnt. This could be applied to contexts wider than language and may facilitate increased confidence.

Child R: Aged seven, attending a language resource
The following is an excerpt from the findings of a DA:

> R's spontaneous language is poorly formulated, but the content is more relevant and understandable than the standardised test scores would suggest. His greatest difficulties lie in the unplanned and impulsive nature of his responses, which interfere with his processing of incoming information and his formulation of language.
>
> His performance on tests is erratic, unpredictable and minimally useful.
>
> R is highly stimulable and responsive to mediation. He is able to benefit from strategies to control his behaviour and structure his approach to a task. He understands and remembers the strategies, but struggles to implement them independently. He demonstrated much improved expressive language when encouraged to slow down and plan.
>
> R's primary need is for behavioural control alongside language therapy.

It can be seen from the examples that information is revealed in the DA relating to the relative strengths of language and non-linguistic cognitive skills. Recommendations for intervention are linked directly to the findings of assessment.

During the trials of the DASS (Hasson 2011), the content of intervention was not controlled. SLTs working with children enrolled in the DA trial were asked to identify broadly the aims of their intervention. They were supplied with reports of the results of the DA.

Without instruction, in response to the information provided, SLTs spontaneously altered their interventions slightly, reducing the emphasis on skills-based therapy and increasing metalinguistic and metacognitive activities.

Monitoring of the children involved in research into the DASS over a period of time revealed that approximately one-third of the children were making little progress in therapy (Hasson 2011). It was this group of children who were shown to make significant gains when their therapy was modified according to the results of the DA. It may be that the value of the DA lies in more detailed assessment and analysis of children who are not responding well to language therapy, but more controlled research is needed into this theory.

A detailed case study that exemplifies the modification of targets informed by the DASS, and subsequent improvements made by the child, was published by Hasson and Dodd (2014).

Reporting of a DA

As the body of research into DA has largely been carried out by EPs, research into the reporting of the results of a DA are based on DA of intelligence and the relationship to school performance. Like Haywood and Lidz (2007), others have explored how a DA may be reported in a school report or incorporated into an Individualized Education Program (IEP).

The difficulty lies in the reporting of a procedure that is unfamiliar to teachers, other EPs and indeed the majority of SLTs. Reports will always need to contain a description of the (dynamic) test; however, Bosma and Resing (2010) found that the responses of teachers to the reports of a DA varied with age and experience, and concluded that reports may also need to contain information about the theory of DA in order to give the readers some context for understanding the information. Deutsch and Reynolds (2000) also pointed out that "clarity of communication is especially important since assessment and intervention are seen as aspects of a single process", which contrasts significantly with the static test.

All of the authors have commented that the findings of a DA can usefully be incorporated into a student's IEP or equivalent. In doing so, it is important to specify the roles of the multidisciplinary team in implementing goals, as the recommendations of the DA are domain general and apply to general cognitive learning principles outside of the area traditionally viewed as SLT. As Deutsch and Reynolds (2000) point out, there is no point in carrying out a DA if the recommendations are not to be implemented.

The reports written about children after their participation in research relating to the DASS followed a fixed format. The reports were made available in the first instance to the SLTs working with the children, who had initially referred them for the study. The SLTs were provided with the following information in advance, which notified them of the data that the DA would elicit:

The information derived from the DA consists of:

- learning needs, for example whether the individual requires metacognitive monitoring, strategy training or item-specific application of knowledge; and
- the individual's learning needs in terms of amount of input required from the examiner.

In addition,

- detail of the language structures that the child has difficulty with, that is additional to that obtained from standardised tests;
- the effect of the amount of content and the nature of semantic content on the child's construction of linguistic structures;
- the child's ability to transfer, or generalise, learning or strategies i.e. item – to item transfer;

- the child's metalinguistic knowledge, ability to label, explain and manipulate linguistic concepts; and

- the child's metacognitive ability i.e. awareness of the processes and strategies that are used to solve the given task.

The DA will also contribute information about the child's

- attention/activity/emotion while engaged in the presented task;

- motivation/attitude to learning/interest/response to input while engaged in the presented task; and

- use of strategies, including reliance on others for help.

The reports then consisted of the following format:

Findings of the DA

Name. . . X   Date. . .

Observations of language problem-solving skills

1 **Detail of language structures that the child has difficulty with, which is additional to that obtained from the standardised tests**

   For example, X is able to use direct and indirect object in sentence

2 **The effect of the amount of content and nature of semantic content on the child's construction of linguistic structures**

   X is aware of logical semantic relationships, humour and absurdity

3 **The child's ability to transfer, or generalise, learning or strategies – i.e. item – to item transfer**

   For example, X made use of inappropriate strategies, such as "*I used 'is' because it's the smallest word*". He was also unable to transfer strategies to successive items.

4 **The child's metalinguistic knowledge, ability to label, explain and manipulate linguistic concepts**

   For example, X demonstrated good task awareness of the need to 'make a sentence'. He was also able to make judgements, recognised a 'good' sentence, and said '*I made a silly sentence.*'

---

5 The child's metacognitive ability – i.e. awareness of the processes and strategies that are used to solve the given task

For example, X confuses linguistic knowledge with metacognitive awareness – e.g. asked, "How did you know. . .?" Responds with "*I thought is . . . Is the man*".

Also unable to explain why he found the task easy and used the sentence structure to explain "*because I used Mum . . .*"

Behavioural factors

- **attention /activity/ emotion while engaged in the presented task**

  X attended well and willingly throughout the task, and although fidgeting and distracted by wall displays in the room, X was easy to refocus and quickly switched attention back to the task.

- **motivation/attitude to learning/interest/response to input while engaged in the presented task**

  X seemed motivated to solve the items and gained intrinsic reward from completing the task items. He was interested and responsive to mediation.

- **use of strategies, including reliance on others for help**

  X made use of linguistic strategies to formulate sentences and transferred structures both within and between items, but he was not able to recognise or articulate most of these strategies. He willingly accepted help with the task, but did not seek or depend on the tester.

Summary of learning needs

X completed almost all of the task items unassisted and demonstrated good implicit use of grammar. He also showed good semantic awareness and easily recognised and accommodated semantic constraints on his sentences, appreciating the humour in inappropriate sentences.

X was very responsive to mediation of strategy use and contributed his own examples. However, he was unable to reflect on the processes he was using, either from a linguistic or cognitive perspective. Vocabulary has not been tested, but X grasped words and tried to use them – e.g. apostrophe, verb. He does not, however, have sufficient metalinguistic knowledge to do this, and cannot explain or justify his grammatical judgements. This will limit his self-monitoring and his access to any higher-level language learning.

X has improved significantly since the previous test, suggesting susceptibility to practice effects, but also a good learning potential. His sentence recall was excellent, which is unusual in children with language disorders.

Recommendations

The recommendation would be to try and further facilitate X's language and communication via mediation of metalinguistic knowledge and reflection. The use of Colourful Semantics would be recommended to help X to recognise, label and manipulate sentence components, and give him tools for reflection on language structure. As X also responded very well to metacognitive ideas, it would seem that he could benefit from further reflection on processes such as planning, relating new information to previous knowledge, hypothetical thinking and justifying his thoughts, as well as maximising his apparent motivation to problem solve (at least in a 1:1 situation).

A template for reporting of the DASS may be found in Appendix A08, and for other DA formats can be found in Appendix B11.

References

Bosma, T., and Resing, W. (2010) 'Teacher's appraisal of dynamic assessment outcomes: Recommendations for weak mathematics performers', *Journal of Cognitive Education and Psychology*, 9(2), pp. 91–115.

Deutsch, R., and Reynolds, Y. (2000) 'The use of dynamic assessment by educational psychologists in the UK', *Educational Psychology in Practice*, 16(3), pp. 311–331.

Feuerstein, R., Feuerstein, R.S., Falik, L.H. and Rand, Y. (2002) *The dynamic assessment of cognitive modifiability: The learning propensity assessment device: Theory, instruments and techniques*, ICELP Press, Jerusalem.

Gopnik, M., and Crago, M.B. (1991) 'Familial aggregation of a developmental language disorder', *Cognition*, 39(1), pp. 1–50.

Hasson, N. (2011). *Dynamic assessment and informed intervention for children with language impairment.* (Unpublished Doctoral thesis) City University London. Online, http://openaccess.city.ac.uk/1119/

Hasson, N., and Dodd, B. (2014) 'Planning intervention using dynamic assessments: A case study', *Child Language Teaching and Therapy*, 30(3), pp. 353–366.

Haywood, H.C., and Lidz, C.S. (2007) *Dynamic assessment in practice: Clinical and educational applications*, Cambridge University Press, New York.

Leonard, L.B. (1998) *Children with specific language impairment*, MIT Press, Cambridge, MA.

Marton, K., and Schwartz, R.G. (2003) 'Working memory capacity and language processes in children with specific language impairment', *Journal of Speech, Language, and Hearing Research*, 46(5), pp. 1138–1154.

Peña, E.D., and Gillam, R.B. (2000) 'Dynamic assessment of children referred for speech and language evaluations', Lidz, C.S., and Elliott, J. (eds) *Dynamic assessment: Prevailing models and applications*, Elsevier Science, Amsterdam.

Appendix A

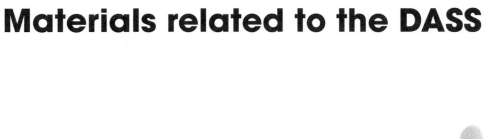
Materials related to the DASS

DASS test items

The full list of test items in versions A and B for reference.

Item	Version A	Version B
1	The boy is washing the car	The girl is reading the book
2	Mary is going to draw a picture	Sue is going to see a film
3	Mum is eating and Dad is drinking	Sara is sitting and Jeni is standing
4	Mum is driving the car and Dad is riding the bike	Lee is pouring the tea and Mum is cutting the cake
5	Jack and Jane fed the baby a bottle	Ben and Sam gave the dog a bone
6	The boy gave the girl a biscuit and a drink	The man showed the boy a bat and a ball
7	The big boy is last	The little girl is late
8	The dog's leg isn't hurt	The cat's face isn't dirty
9	Susie will hide under the table	Marc will look under the bed
10	You can hang your coat on the hook	You can put your keys on the table
11	Joe brushes his teeth before he goes to bed	Holly goes to school after she combs her hair
12	Debby cried because the window broke	Cassie screamed because the door banged

DASS materials set A

the

washing

car

the

is

boy

DASS materials set A.1

a

going

to

draw

is

picture

Mary

DASS materials set A.2

Dad

Mum

is

is

eating

and

drinking

DASS materials set A.3

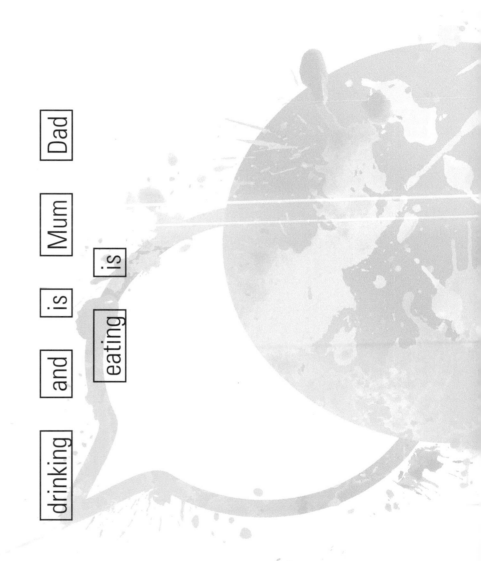

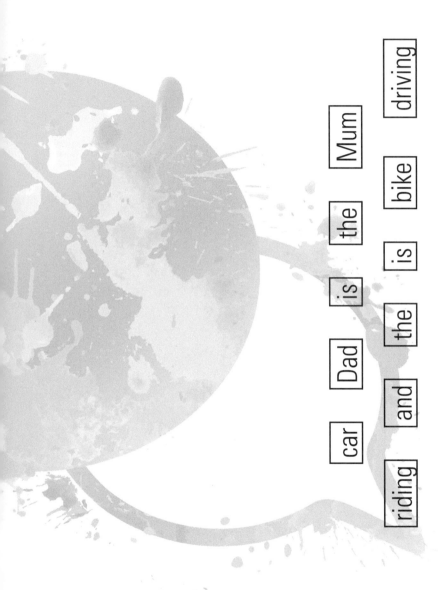

Mum   the   is   Dad   car

driving   bike   is   the   and   riding

DASS materials set A.4

Jack

Jane fed

a the

and baby

bottle

DASS materials set A.5

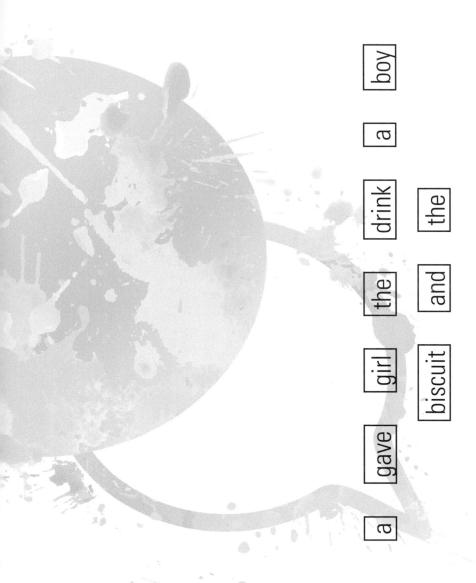

boy

a

drink

the

the

and

girl

biscuit

gave

a

DASS materials set A.6

is

big

last

the

boy

DASS materials set A.7

the

dog's

hurt

leg

isn't

DASS materials set A.8

table

the

hide   Susie

under

will

DASS materials set A.9

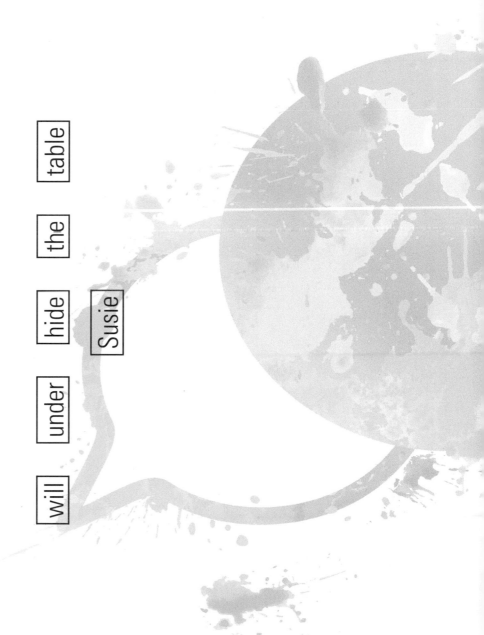

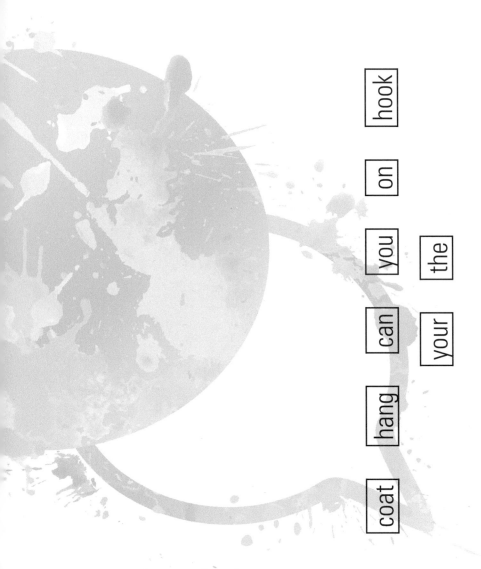

hook

on

you   the

can   your

hang

coat

DASS materials set A.10

teeth

brushes

he

Joe

to

his

before

goes

bed

DASS materials set A.11

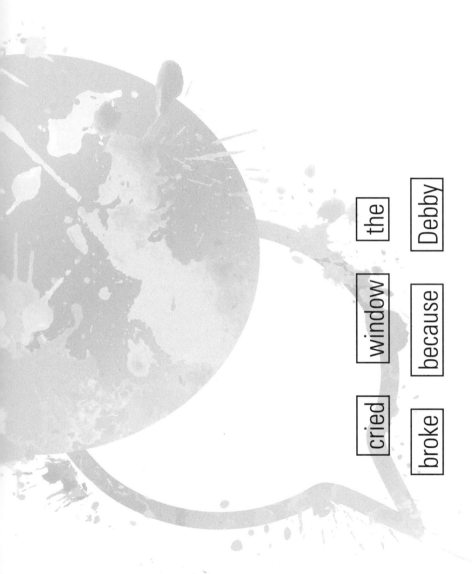

the

Debby

window

because

cried

broke

DASS materials set A.12

DASS materials set B

the

reading

book

the

is

girl

DASS materials set B.1

a

going

to

see

is

film

Sue

DASS materials set B.2

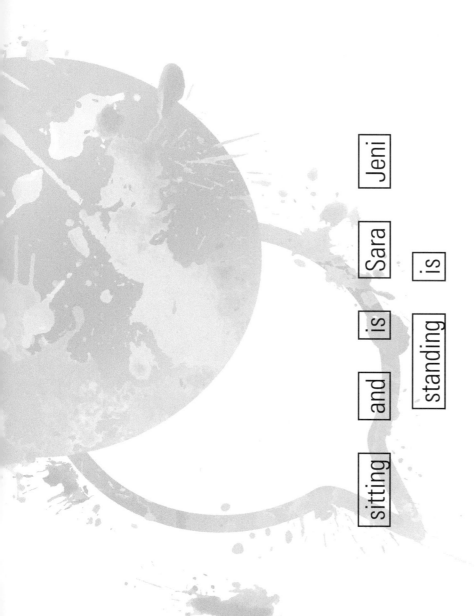

Jeni

Sara is

is and standing

sitting

DASS materials set B.3

cutting

Mum tea

is

the the

is and

Lee pouring

cake

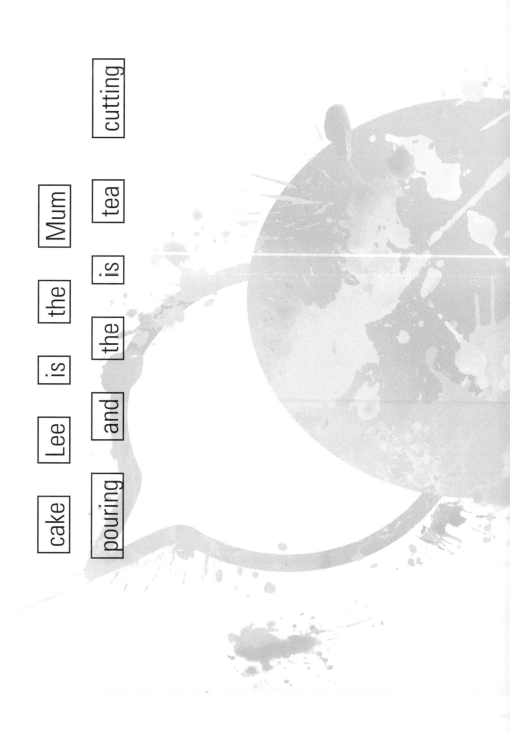

Sam | the | gave | dog | bone

Ben | a | and

DASS materials set B.5

a

bat

the

the

and

boy

ball

showed

man

a

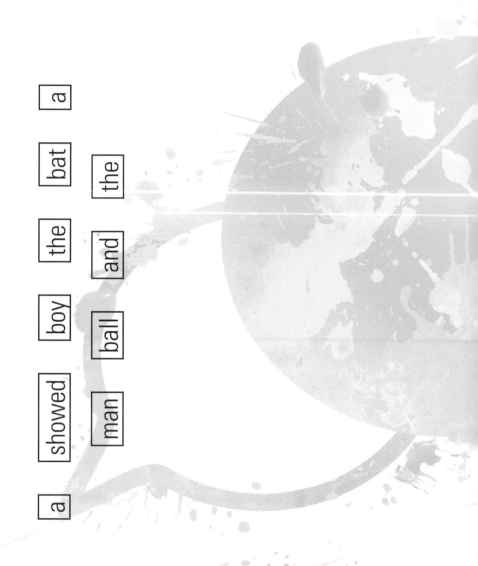

DASS materials set B.6

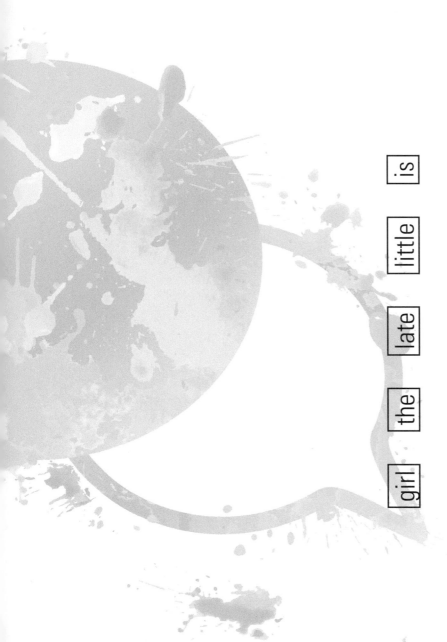

is

little

late

the

girl

DASS materials set B.7

the

cat's

dirty

face

isn't

DASS materials set B.8

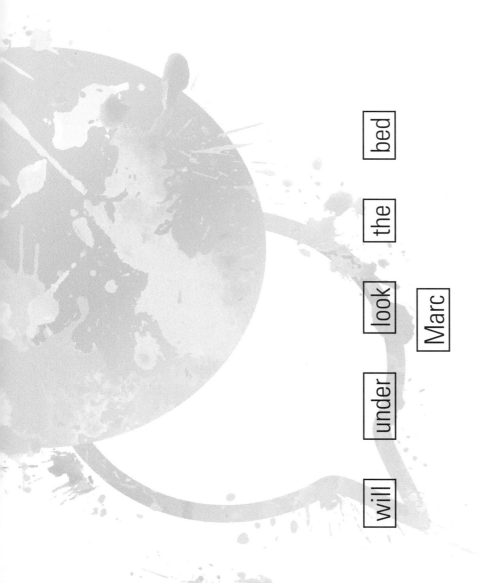

bed

the

look   Marc

under

will

DASS materials set B.9

on

you the

can your

put table

keys

DASS materials set B.10

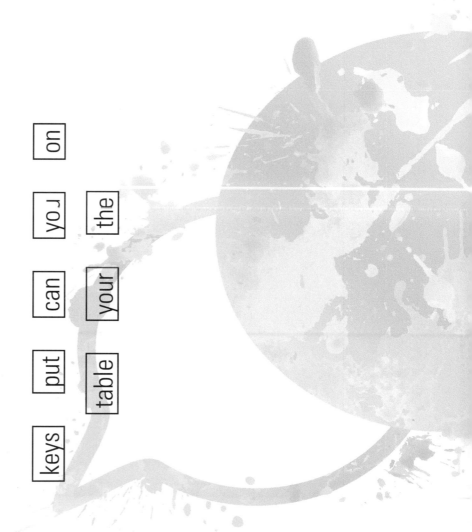

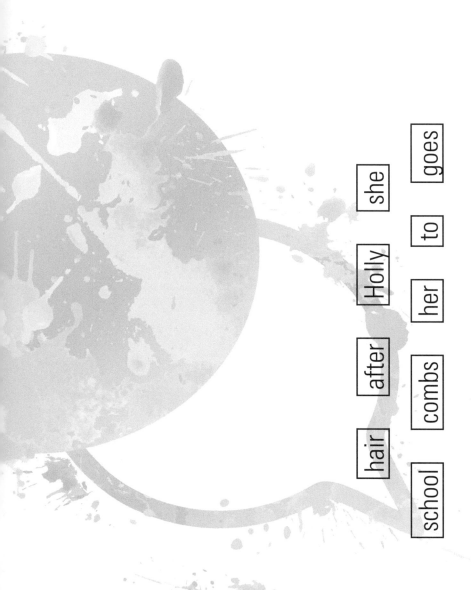

she Holly after hair

to her combs

goes

school

DASS materials set B.11

banged

the Cassie

door because

screamed

DASS materials set B.12

The grammatical structure of DASS items

Item	Structure	Description	Example
1	SVO	Declarative with auxiliary plus main verb	The boy is washing the car
2	SVO	Declarative with auxiliary plus main verb + future tense VP	Mary is going to draw a picture
3	SVcSV	Declarative with coordination	Mum is eating and Dad is drinking
4	SVOcSVO	Declarative with coordination	Mum is driving the car, and Dad is riding the bike
5	SVOdOi	Dative N and N in subject position	Jack and Jane fed the baby a bottle
6	SVOiOd	Dative N and N in object position	The boy gave the girl a biscuit and a drink
7	SVA	Declarative with copula verb and adjective NP	The big boy is last
8	SVA	Declarative with copula verb + contracted negative verb	The dog's leg isn't hurt
9	SVA	Declarative with modal auxiliary plus main verb and prepositional phrase	Susie will hide under the table
10	SVOA	Declarative with modal auxiliary plus main verb, object and prepositional adverbial phrase	You can hang your coat on the hook
11	SVOsSVO	Declarative with subordinate clause (use of anaphoric pronoun)	Joe brushes his teeth before he goes to bed
12	SVsSV	Declarative with subordinate clause	Debby cried because the window broke

Key: S = subject, V = verb, O = object, A = adverbial clause, c = co-ordinating conjunction, s = subordinating conjunction, Od = direct object, Oi = indirect object

Reprinted with permission. Hasson N., Dodd B. & Botting N. (2012) 'Dynamic Assessment of Sentence Structure (DASS): Design and Evaluation of a Novel Procedure for Assessment of Syntax in Children with Language Impairments', *International Journal of Language and Communication Disorders* 47(3), 285–299

Prompt sheet for administration of DASS

1	Spontaneous response	Do you know what you have to do?
2	Drawing on previous knowledge	How did you do this before? Do you know all the words? Is that right? Can you fix it?
3	Finding strategies Problem solving	Which one can you start with? Can you make little groups of words? Can you make a question? Can you swap the words around? Have you used all the words? What have you left out? Reminder: Last time you said. . .
4	Breaking down the task Using specific feedback	Which one can you start with? Which one can you start with to make a question? Start with x. What comes next? You've left this one out. Where does it go? Repeat part of the answer already used. Giving part of the answer.
5	Learning from feedback and instruction	Scaffold sentence bit by bit. Present cloze task. Explain. Identify the errors. Model for imitation.
	Reflection – when the answer is correct	Do you know what you have to do? Is that the right answer? Why was it not OK? Can you tell me how you did that? Was it easy or hard? Why?

Reprinted with permission. **Hasson N., Dodd B. & Botting N.** (2012) 'Dynamic Assessment of Sentence Structure (DASS): Design and Evaluation of a Novel Procedure for Assessment of Syntax in Children with Language Impairments', *International Journal of Language and Communication Disorders* 47(3), 285–299

Scoresheet set A (for use during the DA session)

SET A .... Name.................... Date....................

Item no.	Content structure	Cue 1	Level 2	3	4	5	No. of cues
1a	The boy is washing the car.						
1b	Is the boy washing the car?						
2a	Mary is going to draw a picture.						
2b	Is Mary going to draw a picture?						
3a	Mum is eating, and Dad is drinking.						
3b	(Reversible content)						
4a	Mum is driving the car, and Dad is riding the bike.						
4b	Mum is riding the bike, and Dad is driving the car.						
5a	Jack and Jane fed the baby a bottle.						
5b	Jane and Jack fed the baby a bottle.						
6a	The boy gave the girl a drink and a biscuit.						
6b	(Reversible content)						
7a	The big boy is last.						
7b	Is the big boy last?						
8a	The dog's leg isn't hurt.						
8b	Isn't the dog's leg hurt?						
9a	Susie will hide under the table.						
9b	Will Susie hide under the table?						
10a	You can hang your coat on the hook.						
10b	Can you hang your coat on the hook?						
11a	Joe brushes his teeth before he goes to bed.						
11b	Before he goes to bed, Joe brushes his teeth.						
12a	Debbie cried because the window broke.						
12b	Because the window broke, Debbie cried.						

Total number of cues:_____

Scoresheet set B (for use during the DA session)

SET B ....

Name ....

Date ....

Item no.	Content structure	Cue 1	Level 2	3	4	5	No. of cues
1a	The girl is reading the book.						
1b	Is the girl reading the book?						
2a	Sue is going to see a film.						
2b	Is Sue going to see a film?						
3a	Sara is sitting, and Jeni is standing.						
3b	(Reversible content)						
4a	Lee is pouring the tea, and Mum is cutting the cake.						
4b	Mum is cutting the cake, and Lee is pouring the tea.						
5a	Ben and Sam gave the dog a bone.						
5b	Sam and Ben gave the dog a bone.						
6a	The man showed the boy a bat and a ball.						
6b	(Reversible content)						
7a	The little girl is late.						
7b	Is the little girl late?						
8a	The cat's face isn't dirty.						
8b	Isn't the cat's face dirty?						
9a	Marc will look under the bed.						
9b	Will Marc look under the bed?						
10a	You can put your keys on the table.						
10b	Can you put your keys on the table?						
11a	Holly goes to school after she combs her hair.						
11b	After she combs her hair, Holly goes to school.						
12a	Cassie screamed because the door banged.						
12b	Because the door banged, Cassie screamed.						

Total number of cues:_____

Template for DASS report

Name ....   Date ....

Assessor ....   Place ....

The child was assessed using the The Dynamic Assessment of Sentence Structure (DASS) (Hasson, Dodd and Botting 2012). A dynamic test is one that helps the child with prompts and cues throughout the test in order to assess the child's potential to learn from the practice of doing the test items and from the assistance of the examiner. It enables the examiner to find out not only what language structures are difficult for the child but also what he understands about the structure of sentences, how he approaches a difficult task and what kind of cues help him to succeed.

In the DASS, the child is required to form two different sentences from a set of words presented in a random order. One sentence may be a question, or the order of words may be reversible.

Findings of the dynamic assessment
Observations of language problem-solving skills

1 *Detail of language structures that the child has difficulty with, which is additional to that obtained from the standardised tests.*

2 *The effect of the amount of content and nature of semantic content on the child's construction of linguistic structures.*

3 *The child's ability to transfer, or generalise, learning or strategies – i.e. item – to item transfer.*

4 *The child's metalinguistic knowledge, ability to label, explain and manipulate linguistic concepts.*

5 *The child's metacognitive ability – i.e. awareness of the processes and strategies that are used to solve the given task.*

Behavioural factors

1   *Attention /activity/ emotion while engaged in the presented task*

2   *Motivation/attitude to learning/interest/response to input while engaged in the presented task*

3   *Use of strategies, including reliance on others for help*

Summary of learning needs

Recommendations

_____

Appendix B

Supplementary materials

Required mediational intervention

This scale, devised by Feuerstein *et al.* (2002 p. 533), can be used to score the level of cues required to facilitate problem solving by the individual.

Examples of its application to language tasks are added alongside.

LOW LEVELS OF DISTANCE/HIGHER DEGREE OF MANIFEST RMI			
Distance level	Examiner	Examinee	Examples from SLT interventions
0	Produces response via direct imposition on examinee	*Passive*, conforms to pressure of examiner to reproduce model	Direct imitation, mouthing/pointing response alongside child
1	Models act to be copied, encourages imitation, withdraws as examinee starts to respond	Aware of mediator's intervention, initiates partially successful representation of model	Direct model, model of part of utterance, a cloze task or model with a choice of items for completion
2	Points out specific examples of rules, concepts, attributes of the problem, identifies constant and changing elements	Spontaneously responds to task, attends to mediator's verbal and motor intervention	Uses specific example to demonstrate types of words or elements of sentence. *This one is a boy, this one a girl. Is this happening now, or is it already done?*
3	Identifies general class characteristics	Encouraged to apply response to repeated or varied situation	*Can you identify the verb? Question word?*
MIDDLE LEVELS OF DISTANCE/MODERATE AND VARIABLE DEGREE OF MEDIATION			
4	Refers to previously identified strategies	Acts on previous mediation, applies and repeats, no rules formulated	*What do you do first/next? What do we look for?*

(*Continued*)

(Continued)

MIDDLE LEVELS OF DISTANCE/MODERATE AND VARIABLE DEGREE OF MEDIATION			
Distance level	Examiner	Examinee	Examples from SLT interventions
5	Selects/encourages strategies based on insight and rules	Chooses adequate strategies based on derived insight	Look carefully at all of the words. Have you left anything out?
6	Points out previously used strategies using transcending verbal and metalinguistic rules	Applies previously used strategies, reflects awareness of rules and operations	We need to make a plan. What are the rules?
HIGHER LEVELS OF DISTANCE/LOWER DEGREE OF RMI			
7	Focuses examinee attention on problem anticipatory, and pre-response mediation, to provide initial regulation of response	Formulates specific rules, strategies, attitudes and meanings, self-regulatory	Are you ready? You may have to remember what you used before
8	Alerts to metacognitive elements, directs mediation to structural change, challenges for resistance and flexibility	Elements of structural change consistently present	What have you learnt?
9	Passive presence in elicitation of responses	Mediation is fully internalised, self-regulation	Targets are produced without help.

Reprinted with permission. Feuerstein R., Feuerstein R. S., Falik L. H. & Rand Y. (2002) *The Dynamic Assessment of Cognitive Modifiability: The Learning Propensity Assessment Device: Theory, Instruments and Techniques*, ICELP Press, Jerusalem

Prompt hierarchy for phonological analysis tasks

This schema may be adapted for use with a range of PA tasks, as described in Chapter 3

	Prompt type	Example of prompt
1.	Instructions	Do you know what you have to do? Can you tell me?
2.	Preparation	Do you know what all the words mean?
		Give me an example of one
		Can you read these materials?
3.	Cognitive strategies	Have you done this before?
		Do you remember what you did before?
		Let's make a plan for this
		What do you need to do first? Why?
		What would be a good/better way to do this?
4.	Task specific	Can you break this up into parts?
		Is there something we need to change? What?
		Would it help to write this down? Or draw something?
		Is there a rule that would help us?
5.	Item specific	We have this and this.
		Now do this to it.
		Does that work?
	Transfer	Can you do the same again?
	Reflection	Is that right?
		How do you know?
		Was that difficult? Why?

Prompt hierarchy for morphological analysis tasks

This schema may be used for a variety of structures with morphological endings as described in Chapter 3.

For example, "Here is a wug. Now there are two. There are two. . . ?"

"This dog likes to walk. Every day he . . . ?" " Yesterday he . . . ?"

	Prompt type	Example of prompt
1.	Instructions	Do you know what you have to do? Can you tell me?
2.	Preparation	Can you read these materials?
		Do you know this word (or picture), or do you think it might be something made-up?
		Can you show me the *beginning* of this word?
		And the *ending*?
		When might we put something on the end of a word?
		What might we put on the end of a word?
		Is there a rule that would help us?
3.	Cognitive strategies	Have you done this before?
		Do you remember what you did before?
		Can you think of something that sounds like this word?
		Can you use any rules that you know?
		What would be a good/better way to do this?
4.	Task specific	Can you see if this word (e.g. cars/houses/walks/walked) has an ending added on? What about this one (e.g. hand/walk – root word only)?
		Can you break this word (e.g. shoes/painted) up into parts?
		What does this part (-s/es/ed ending) mean?
		Would it help to write this down?
5.	Item specific	Here we have one of these, and here we have two.
		If we have a dog, and then two we say two dogs.
		So if we have one wug, then we have two. Wug plus -s

Prompt type	Example of prompt
Transfer	Can you do the same again?
Reflection	Is that right?
	How do you know?
	Was that difficult? Why?

DA of Morphological analysis

This can be used with morphologically complex words from the national curriculum, as described in Chapter 3.

Hasson N, Nash L, Cubie B, Kessie A & Marshall C (2014) *Dynamic assessment of morphological analysis: A UK based Study.* Poster presented to RCSLT Conference, University of Leeds.

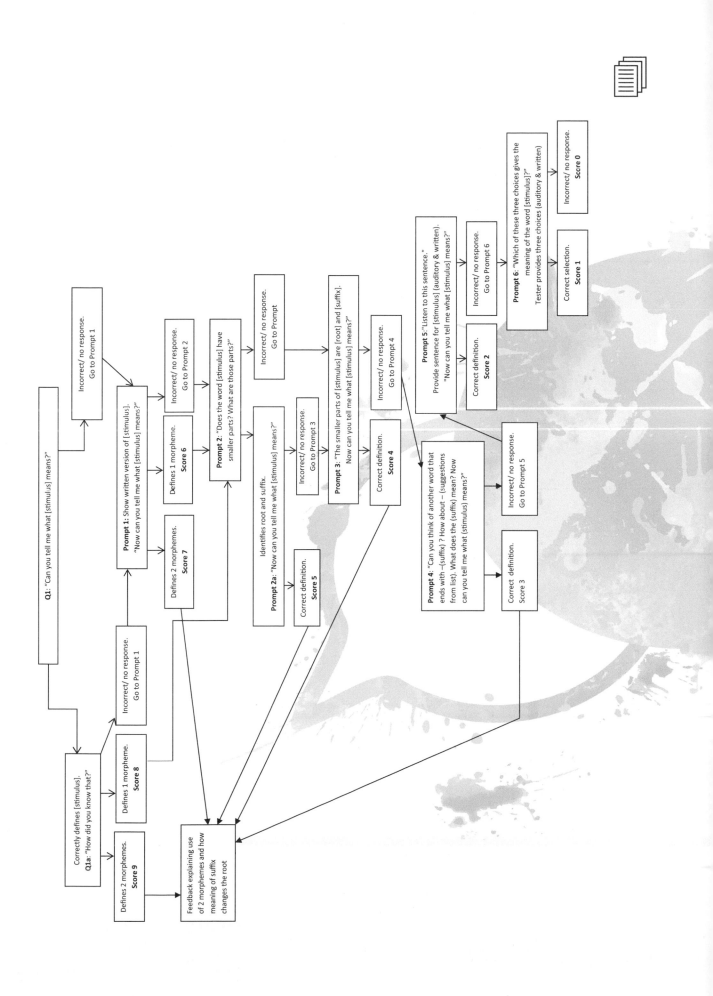

Q1: "Can you tell me what [stimulus] means?"

Incorrect/ no response. Go to Prompt 1

Correctly defines [stimulus]. **Q1a:** "How did you know that?"

Defines 1 morpheme. **Score 8**

Defines 2 morphemes. **Score 9**

Incorrect/ no response. Go to Prompt 1

Prompt 1: Show written version of [stimulus]. "Now can you tell me what [stimulus] means?"

Incorrect/ no response. Go to Prompt 2

Defines 1 morpheme. **Score 6**

Defines 2 morphemes. **Score 7**

Prompt 2: "Does the word [stimulus] have smaller parts? What are those parts?"

Incorrect/ no response. Go to Prompt

Identifies root and suffix. **Prompt 2a:** "Now can you tell me what [stimulus] means?"

Incorrect/ no response. Go to Prompt 3

Correct definition. **Score 5**

Prompt 3: "The smaller parts of [stimulus] are [root] and [suffix]. Now can you tell me what [stimulus] means?"

Incorrect/ no response. Go to Prompt 4

Correct definition. **Score 4**

Prompt 4: "Can you think of another word that ends with –(suffix) ? How about – (suggestions from list). What does the (suffix) mean? Now can you tell me what (stimulus) means?"

Incorrect/ no response. Go to Prompt 5

Correct definition. Score 3

Prompt 5: "Listen to this sentence." Provide sentence for [stimulus] (auditory & written). "Now can you tell me what [stimulus] means?"

Incorrect/ no response. Go to Prompt 6

Correct definition. **Score 2**

Prompt 6: "Which of these three choices gives the meaning of the word [stimulus]?" Tester provides three choices (auditory & written)

Incorrect/ no response. **Score 0**

Correct selection. **Score 1**

Feedback explaining use of 2 morphemes and how meaning of suffix changes the root

Cognitive functions

These cognitive functions, adapted from Feuerstein *et al.* (2002), were considered in the *The use of dynamic methods of language assessment in language impaired children* (Hasson 2005), as described in Chapter 3. The selected cognitive functions were rated on a five-point scale.

Input

- *Systematic and careful gathering of information* (Has the child looked carefully at the stimulus picture and taken in all aspects?)

- *Labelling* (Has he given the things he has seen a name so he can identify them clearly, refer to them and remember them better? This is also an opportunity to ensure that the child has the necessary vocabulary, or supply it as required)

- *Establishing temporal and spatial reference* (Can he describe where and when things occur?)

- *Organisation of information from two sources at the same time* (Can he relate what he sees in the picture to the information being requested in the prompt question?)

Elaboration

- *Defining the problem* (Can he figure out what he is being asked to do?)

- *Relevance* (Can he identify the parts of the information gathered (from the picture) that are important and discard or ignore those which are not needed?)

- *Projecting Relationships* (Can he find relationships that link the items identified?)

- *Planning behaviour* (Can he arrange objects and events into the most logical order to express their relationship to each other?)

Output

- *Planning output* (Can he overcome impulsive and trial-and-error responses?)

- *Overcome egocentric communication* (Can he formulate a clear and precise answer, and make sure the listener will understand?)

- *Overcoming blocking* (Can he use a strategy to answer the question instead of panicking and not answering, or saying I don't know)

Cognitive functions rating scale

Picture No:_____

Cognitive function	1 Very deficient	2 Quite deficient	3 Adequate	4 Quite efficient	5 Very efficient
Input					
Systematic info gathering					
Labelling/verbal tools					
Temporal and spatial reference					
Using two sources of info					
Elaboration					
Defining the problem					
Relevance					
Projecting relationships					
Planning behaviour					
Output					
Planning output					
Overcoming egocentricity					
Overcoming blocking					

Mediation script for DA of narrative

The following script, reprinted with the kind permission of Elizabeth Peña, was used alongside the dynamic test of narrative, (Miller, Gillam & Peña 2001) in one of the sessions of mediated intervention. It refers to one of the storybooks used in the test and may be used as an example of mediated intervention for story structure.

Today we're going to talk about telling complete stories. When people tell stories, they include a number of parts. They tell what the problem is, what the characters did, how they solve the problem and how they feel about that. As you tell the story, let's talk about the characters, where the story takes place and when it takes place.

It's important to be able to tell good stories because children tell each other stories all the time, and you read and write stories in school. So learning to tell complete stories helps you communicate better and do better in school. Now why is it important to tell better stories? [Help child to explain that stories are important for school and for communication.]

First, let's talk about the different parts that need to be in a story. Storytellers start their stories by telling when and where something happened. That helps us understand the world the character lives in. So what do we need to think about when we start a story [when and where or setting]?

[Refer to p. 1 in Two Friends] How does this story start [pause, wait for response, help child to respond when needed]? Where do you think they are [pause, wait for response]? What time do you think it is [pause, wait for response]? How would you start a story in a way that tells where and when the story takes place? [Pause, let them fill in, if they don't, give an example such as "one morning the dog and cat stood by the river" that tells us when and where.]

We also need to know about the characters. Good storytellers tell listeners about who the characters are and what they're like. We also need to include what [character information]? Let's think about the characters. What do they look like [pause, wait for response]? Do the dog and the cat have names [pause, wait for response]? You could say Bill the dog and Sally the cat were talking about what they were going to do that day. You can also tell what they look like or think of names that describe them. For example, I could say, Triangles, and who would that describe? Yes, the cat. Triangles the cat was thinking about. . . [can additionally use toys or puppets to name/describe].

In stories, we also want to talk about what happened first, second and last, and why things happened (order and causal relationships). This is important because it helps us understand the order of the story and the reasons the characters (people) did what they did.

What would happen if you told the story backwards or out of order? [Help child state that it would be hard to know what happened when, or that it would be hard to know why it happened.] At the beginning of the story, first, they were. . . [help child to describe] and then [turn page] [help child describe]. We use words like first, next and then to describe what happened and why it happened (order and causal relationships) [using puppets, let child act out the story and explain the order and causal relationships].

Let's tell a story that includes all these pieces [help child tell story with setting, time, place, characters, temporal order and causality] [Wow, that was good] [Example: Triangles the cat and Rex the dog were standing by the river talking. While they were talking, Rex fell asleep. So Triangles left because she had no one to talk to]. In this story, you remembered to include. . . [list what they included].

Always remember to talk about the setting (when and where), character information, order (temporal) and causal relationships. In this story, what is the setting [let child fill in, assist him]? What should we say about the characters [let child fill in, assist him]? What happened first? Then what? Then what [let child fill in, assist him]? And why did the cat leave? Why did the dog look for the cat [let child fill in, assist him]? It's important to include these things because they tell us about the world the characters live in (setting), the order of the story (order) and the reasons the characters did what they did (causal relationships).

Tell me what these are again. Character information [let child respond, assist if necessary], setting (when and where) [let child respond, assist if necessary], order (temporal) [let child respond, assist if necessary] and causal relationships [let child respond, assist if necessary].

Next, we're going to talk about telling complete stories. When people tell stories, they include a beginning, a middle and an end. They tell what the problem is at the beginning and how the characters feel about the problem. For the middle, they talk about the actions the characters take to solve the problem. At the end, they talk about how the characters eventually solved the problem and how they feel once the problem is solved.

Do you remember why stories are important [Expand on what child says – e.g. it's important to be able to tell good stories because children tell each other stories all the time, and you read and write stories in school. So learning to tell complete stories helps you communicate better and to do better in school.]

Let's talk about the different parts that need to be in a story. When people tell stories, they need to know what happened to start the action in the story. This is called a problem. What do we need to include? [Problem]. [Refer to p. 1 in Two Friends] How does this story start? [child answers] [turn the page] What do you think caused the problem? [let them fill in] To include the problem, you would say. . . [pause, let them fill it in, if they don't give example "One morning, the cat and the dog were talking and the dog fell asleep, that tells us what started the problem".] [reflect what he said – use expansion/extension as needed] [let child act out with puppets.]

After the problem we talk about how the character feels about it. That is important because it makes the story interesting and helps us understand why they did things. What happens to the dog on this page (page 2)? Yes, he falls asleep. That's the problem. Over here (page 3), how does the cat feel about the dog falling asleep? Ok, so what are we calling them? [then continue using the names selected] Right, Sally is sad because Bill fell asleep. Why do you think she felt sad? [Yes, Sally feels sad because Bill didn't want to talk to her anymore.] What do you think she said to Bill? [Hey Bill, wake up and talk to me.] But, did he wake up? [No, even though Sally tried to wake him up, he didn't.] So (page 4) what does Sally do? [wait for child response] Yes. When Bill wouldn't wake up, Sally decided to leave. You need to include how characters feel about what happened.

After we talk about how characters feel, we talk about how they try to solve the problem. We also need to include what [the attempts]. [Refer to p. 8 in Two Friends] What does the dog do? [Pause. Let him fill it in; if he doesn't, give an example "He asks the animals if they have seen the cat".]

After we talk about what the character does, we need to tell how the problem was solved. What happened after the dog looked for the cat? [Child responds that the dog found the cat]. That's right; what was the problem [the cat was gone]? And how did the dog solve the problem [he looked for the cat and he found it]?

After talking about how the problem was solved, storytellers can tell how the characters feel about it or their reaction. How did the story end? [Pause. Let him fill it in; if he doesn't, give the example "The dog and the cat became friends again".] Do you think they were happy? How would you feel? Why?

Stories include problems, the way people feel about them, what they do to try to solve them, what happens and how they feel at the end. Why is this important? [This is important because it helps your friends understand your story and helps you do better in school.] I want you to tell me the story of the Two Friends again [let child use puppets to tell the story if he chooses].

How are you going to remember to tell a complete story with all the different parts? [Discuss strategies to include specific components of story and a complete episode.]

Mediated learning experience rating scale

This scale, reprinted with permission from Lidz C.S. (1991) *Practitioner's Guide to Dynamic Assessment.* **The Guilford Press, New York, is used to capture the use of mediational behaviours by an assessor. It is described in Chapter 4.**

1   INTENTIONALITY: a conscious attempt by the mediator to influence the behavior of the child. This includes communication to the child of the purpose for the interaction, as well as attempts by the mediator to maintain the child's involvement in the interaction. For children who are already self-regulating and do not require interventions by the mediator to engage them in the activity, rating of intentionality includes the readiness of the mediator to become involved as necessary; therefore, the mediator shows ongoing interest in the active involvement of the child (Assign 2 in this case).

    0 = no evidence

    1 = inconsistently present; loses involvement

    2 = consistently in evidence

    3 = in evidence with statement or encouragement of a principle to induce self-regulation in the child; this principle would apply to the child's ability to maintain attention and inhibit impulsivity.

    NOTES:

2   MEANING: moving the content from neutral to a position of value and importance; this may be done by affective emphasis, gesture, movement of the materials, or by stating that the object or aspect of focus is important and should be noticed (or vice versa, that it is negative and to be ignored or avoided).

    0 = not in evidence

    1 = calling up labels or concepts already within the child's repertory; saying that it is important and should be noticed (e.g. "look at this") but without elaboration

    2 = adding animation or affect to make the activity come alive and provoke interest

    3 = elaboration that expands the information about the activity or object or that provides information about the cultural meaning or relevance

    NOTES:

3 TRANSCENDENCE: promotion of cognitive bridges between the task or activity and related but not currently present experiences of the child; these may refer to the past or may anticipate the future. This must promote visual images and help to move the child from the perceptual to the conceptual, that is, to what the child can not now see.

0 = not in evidence

1 = simple, non-elaborated reference to past or future experience

2 = elaborated reference

3 = elaborated reference includes hypothetical, inferential, or cause/effect thinking

NOTES:

4 JOINT REGARD: looking and/or commenting on an object of focus initiated by the child; this also includes trying (figuratively or literally) to 'see' the activity from the child's point of view, for example, changing posture or making a comment to express empathy and state a feeling or thought that the child might be experiencing. Finally, this also includes statements expressing the 'we-ness' of the experience, as in using the term 'let's. . .' – for example, "Wow, that was really hard; we had to work a long time to figure that one out!"

0 = not in evidence

1 = clear occurrence, but unelaborated reference

2 = simple elaboration

3 = helping the child express a thought that the child was otherwise unable to elaborate; the expression of the thought should appear to be an accurate reflection of the child's thinking or feeling

NOTES:

5 SHARING OF EXPERIENCE/THOUGHT: communication to the child of an experience or thought the mediator had that the child had not previously shared or experienced with the mediator. For example, comments including "When I was a little girl . . .", or "This makes me think of . . ." should relate to the activity being shared.

0 = not in evidence

1 = clear, but non-elaborated reference

2 = elaborated reference

3 = elaborated reference includes hypothetical, cause/effect or inferential thinking

NOTES:

6 TASK REGULATION: promoting competence through manipulation of the task to facilitate mastery by the child.

0 = not in evidence

1 = simple directions or passive manipulation of the task – e.g. holding it, moving pieces towards the child

2 = elaborated directions or non-verbal organisation into a kind of conceptual grouping

3 = induction/statement/encouragement or strategic thinking and a planning attitude, e.g. "Where shall we start?" "What should we do first?" The mediator can be rated a (3) also if there is statement of a principle that the child can use to solve similar problems

NOTES:

7   PRAISE/ENCOURAGEMENT: promoting competence through verbal or non-verbal communication to the child that s/he did a good job. (Deduct one point for negative, put-down remarks – i.e. one total point for each remark.)

0 = not in evidence

1 = occasional display of non-verbal touch/hug; occasional statement of good, fine, right . . .

2 = frequent displays of non-verbal touch/hug or frequent statements of good, fine, right . . . (frequent = three or more) (two points are also given if the mediator provides encouraging remarks in an attempt to help preserve the child's self-esteem, even if these are not clear praise)

3 = occasional or frequent praise includes information about the child's performance that seemed to help the child – e.g. "You really looked at all the choices; that was great!"

NOTES:

8   CREATING A CHALLENGE ZONE: (for application to teachers and assessors; may be omitted for parents for short interactions). Promoting competence through creating a challenge zone involves maintenance of the activity or task within the child's "zone of proximal [or next] development" – i.e. neither too high nor too low for the child's ability to deal with the task demands; the child should be challenged to reach beyond the current level of functioning, but not so overwhelmed as to be discouraged from attempts to engage in the task.

0 = not in evidence or activity is overly frustrating or much too below the level of challenge

1 = some success in accurate maintenance within the child's range; inconsistently maintained

2 = generally successful; more in evidence than not

3 = general success includes articulation to the child the principle that was involved – e.g. stating that "you really had to think and work hard on this, but you were able to do it with only a little help!" Or, "I want to make this a little hard for you so you have to think, but I'll give you some help so you will know what to do".

NOTES:

9   PSYCHOLOGICAL DIFFERENTIATION: maintenance of the idea that the role of the mediator is to facilitate the learning of the child, not to have a learning experience for oneself (at this

time). Thus, there would be no indications of competitiveness with the child or of rejection of the child's efforts to engage in the task. The focus of the mediator is on provision of a good learning experience rather than on creation of a good product; if something has to be sacrificed, it is the end product, not the child's experience. (1 point is deducted if the mediator rejects the child's efforts to become involved.)

0 = not in evidence; mediator poorly differentiated

1 = activity is mostly mediator's; only occasionally the child's

2 = activity is mostly the child's, with only occasional lapses by the mediator

3 = activity is clearly and consistently child's, with mediator maintaining an objective facilitating role

NOTES:

10 CONTINGENT RESPONSIBILITY: ability to read the child's cues and signals related to learning, affective, and motivational needs, and then respond in a timely and appropriate way.

0 = not in evidence

1 = infrequent, inconsistent (ill-timed or not appropriate)

2 = present, but occasionally misses the mark either in timing or in appropriateness

3 = consistently well timed and appropriate to child's cues and signals

NOTES:

11 AFFECTIVE INVOLVEMENT: communication of a sense of caring about and enjoyment of the child; this may be overt or more quietly covert, but it should be clear that there is a feeling of joy in the child's presence with signs of emotional attachment. This would appear more strongly in a parent compared to teacher or examiner, but should be in evidence in any of the mediators.

0 = not in evidence; indifferent; may be negative

1 = minimal evidence; neutral but not negative or indifferent

2 = clear evidence; may have lapses

3 = clear and consistent enjoyment

NOTES:

12 CHANGE (for application to teachers and assessors): communication to the child that s/he has profited in a positive direction from the experience, that s/he has improved and changed in some way compared to the starting point. This includes providing the child with actual pre-/post-product comparisons, as well as pre-/post-behavioral descriptions.

0 = not in evidence

1 = weak evidence

2 = strong, but unelaborated evidence

3 = strong indications include elaborated feedback regarding what the child did and what the changes were; these might include elicitations from the child regarding what s/he notices has changed

SCORE SEPARATELY AND DO NOT INCLUDE IN MLE TOTAL, BUT INCLUDE FOR ALL ACTIVITIES:

RECIPROCITY OF CHILD:* the level of receptivity of the child to the mediational interactions with the adult; how open is the child to input from the mediator? How able or willing is the child to 'receive' or cooperate?

0 = highly resistant; cannot effectively proceed

1 = minimally receptive; frequent resistance

2 = moderately receptive; occasional lapses

3 = consistently receptive and cooperative

NOTES:

PROFILE OF MEDIATOR FUNCTIONING ON THE MEDIATED LEARNING EXPERIENCE RATING SCALE

	3	*2*	*1*	*0*
1 Intentionality				
2 Meaning				
3 Transcendence				
4 Joint Regard				
5 Sharing of Experiences				
6 Task Regulation				
7 Praise/Encouragement				
8 Challenge				
9 Psychological Differentiation				
10 Contingent Responsivity				
11 Affective Involvement				
12 Change				

Child's Responsivity:

Summary:

Rating scale for mediational behaviours used by speech and language therapists

This scale was devised for the monitoring of the use of mediational techniques by the assessor during a DA. It can be used by practitioners as a self-monitoring tool. See Chapter 4.

Part A

Mediation of intentionality – conveying to the child that you intend to help him improve, 'This includes communication to the child of the purpose for the interaction, as well as attempts by the mediator to maintain the child's involvement in the interaction'.

For example, keeping the child involved.

Statements to child to maintain attention and inhibit impulsivity – e.g. "Read or look carefully at all the words".

PRESENT/ABSENT

Mediation of meaning – sharing the purpose of the activity, 'moving the content from neutral to a position of value and importance'

For example, pointing out labels or concepts known to the child.

Adding animation or affect (or humour) to provoke or maintain interest

Expanding information about the activity

PRESENT/ABSENT

Mediation of transcendence – linking the activity to other contexts in which the skill can be used, 'promotion of cognitive bridges between the task or activity and related but not currently present experiences of the child; these may refer to the past or may anticipate the future'

For example, reference to tasks in the past or future.

Elaborated hypothetical, inferential or cause and effect thinking

PRESENT/ABSENT

Mediation of a feeling of competence – targeting praise so that the child learns what he has done well, learns that the tester has confidence in him, and gains confidence in his own ability.

Praise + Differentiated feedback

PRESENT/ABSENT

Sub score, Part A: /4

◇◇

Part B

1 **Supply the information** that may be needed to learn relationships or find solutions

Explain to child about forming questions, names, verbs, etc.

PRESENT /ABSENT

2 **Ask questions** – i.e. elicit rather than give answers

Asking the child what to do rather than telling him

PRESENT /ABSENT

3 Asking child to evaluate right/wrong rather than telling him

PRESENT /ABSENT

4 Challenge the child to justify his answers, both right and wrong responses

PRESENT /ABSENT

5 Asking child to Bridge to different applications

For example, "When is another time you could do that?"

PRESENT /ABSENT

6 Bring about induction of rules by **calling attention to similarities** among events or examples

"Have you seen one like this before? How did you do it? Does it apply to this?"

PRESENT /ABSENT

7 Facilitate **application of rules and strategic thinking**

For example, which word can we use to start a question/ a statement?

Does it make sense to say Xxx? (e.g. 'a the man')

Reduce trial-and-error behaviour, guessing and random answers.

PRESENT /ABSENT

8 Maintain a metacognitive emphasis – i.e. focus attention on the child's own thinking

processes and encourage them to do the same

Ask process questions – usually containing 'how'.

How did you know? How else could you do that? How can you find out?

How did you do that? What did you do that time? Where did you learn that?

PRESENT /ABSENT

Sub score, Part B: /8

TOTAL SCORE /12

Response to mediation scale

This scale, reproduced with permission from Lidz C.S. (2003) *Early Childhood Assessment*. Wiley, New Jersey, is useful to rate and record the responsiveness of an individual during an assessment session and in interaction with an assessor. It can be used during a variety of activities. See Chapter 4.

RESPONSE TO MEDIATION SCALE

Child:

Date:

A SELF-REGULATION OF ATTENTION

1   Unable to maintain attention to task
2   Fleeting attention to task even with input from adult
3   Maintains with significant input from adult
4   Maintains with occasional input from adult
5   Maintains with no input from adult
    Does not apply

B SELF-REGULATION OF MOTOR ACTIVITY

1   Impulsive to point of disruption
2   Impulsiveness needs significant restraint from adult
3   Impulsive control needs moderate restraint from adult
4   Impulsive control needs minimal restraint from adult
5   No evidence of difficulty with impulse control
    Does not apply

C SELF-REGULATION OF EMOTIONS

1   Extreme emotional lability, difficulty self-calming
2   Significant emotional lability, difficulty self-calming
3   Minimal emotional lability, able to self-calm
4   Rare emotional lability, able to self-calm
5   No evidence of emotional lability
    Does not apply

(Continued)

(Continued)

D STRATEGIC PROBLEM SOLVING

1   Does not engage in any organised manner with task
2   Engages but uses trial-and-error approach
3   Pauses for seeming momentary reflection before proceeding
4   Some evidence of planned and organised task involvement
5   Clearly planned and well-organised approach
    Does not apply

E EVIDENCE OF SELF-TALK WHEN WORKING ON CHALLENGING TASK

1   No evidence
2   Makes noises, but these express effort, not task
3   Verbalises, but content is not task related
4   Makes task-related comments
5   Task-related comments guide efforts at task solution (including muttered, unclear comments)
    Does not apply

F INTERACTIVITY WITH MEDIATOR

1   Does not engage in turntaking communications
2   Minimal engagement in turntaking communications
3   Moderate engagement in turntaking communications
4   Comfortable, frequent engagement in turntaking communications
5   Initiates and responds appropriately and expansively in several chains of conversational interactions
    Does not apply

G RESPONSIVENESS TO INITIATIONS OF MEDIATOR

1   Resistive to mediator's initiatives
2   Passive noncompliant
3   Passive minimally responsive
4   Consistently responsive
5   Enthusiastic and responsive
    Does not apply

H COMPREHENSION OF THE TASK

1   No evidence of task comprehension
2   Willing imitator, but needs model, demonstration or move through
3   Slow to comprehend, but does eventually get it
4   Average comprehension of task
5   Quick to comprehend task
    Does not apply

I RESPONSE TO CHALLENGE

1   Refuses, cries or tantrums in response to challenge
2   Begins but quickly gives up
3   Persists, but with significant encouragement from adult
4   Persists and completes task, with minimal adult encouragement
5   Energised by challenge, enjoys the challenge
    Does not apply

J USE OF ADULT AS A RESOURCE WHEN CHILD NEEDS HELP

1   Does not refer to adult
2   Non-verbally, passively signals need for help
3   Non-verbally actively seeks help
4   Verbally asks for help
5   Actively seeks help and seems to appreciate help provided
    Does not apply

K INTEREST IN ACTIVITY MATERIALS

1   Shows dislike of materials
2   Neutral reaction to materials
3   Minimal interest in materials
4   Fluctuating interest in materials
5   Consistently strong interest in materials
    Does not apply

Mediated learning observation checklist

This scale, reprinted with permission from Elizabeth Peña, was first published in Peña E. D., Resendiz M & Gillam R. B. (2007) 'The Role of Clinical Judgements of Modifiability in the Diagnosis of Language Impairment', *International Journal of Speech-Language Pathology*, 9(4), pp 332–345. It is used to rate the responses of the individual during administration of a task.

	1	*2*	*3*	*4*	*5*
Internal Social-Emotional (Affect)					
Anxiety	Calm, little to no soothing required	Fidgety but can be soothed	Uncomfortable, breaks needed to sooth	Distressed, much soothing required	Distraught, crying, cannot be soothed
Motivation	Enthusiastic, engages in tasks readily	Curious, shows interest	Ambivalent, unsure about tasks	Guarded, seems fearful of tasks	Avoidant, does not want to engage
Non-verbal persistence	Persistent, wants to continue despite difficulty	Indicates difficulty non-verbally, but continues	Tentative, appears unsure about continuing	Demonstrates non-verbal frustration, continues under protest	Non-verbal rejecting, cannot continue
Comments					
Cognitive Arousal					
Task orientation	Completely understands tasks	Mostly understands tasks (75%)	Understands tasks some of the time (50%)	Often does not understand tasks (25% of the time)	Doesn't understand tasks
Metacognition	Aware of all errors	Aware of most errors (75%)	Aware of some errors (50%)	Unaware of most errors (25%)	Unaware of any errors

	1	*2*	*3*	*4*	*5*
Non-verbal self-reward	Positive response to task regardless of difficulty	Positive response related to task difficulty	Demonstrates insecurity, positive and negative responses related to difficulty	Negative response related to task difficulty	Negative response regardless of task difficulty
Comments					

Cognitive Elaboration

	1	*2*	*3*	*4*	*5*
Problem solving	Systematic and efficient, used forethought, reflection	Organised, but somewhat inefficient, (less than 25% of task)	Sketchy plan, trial and error	Disorganised, haphazard plan	No plan; unsystematic guessing
Verbal mediation	Elaborates plan clearly	Talks through problem	Talks occasionally	One- to two-word utterances only	No verbal mediation
Flexibility	Uses multiple strategies readily	Has preferred strategies, but can change when necessary	Some evidence of more than one strategy and occasionally utilises them	Recognises limitation of strategy, but cannot see alternatives	Persists with one strategy, regardless of outcome
Comments					

External Social-Emotional (Behaviour)

	1	*2*	*3*	*4*	*5*
Responsiveness to feedback	Very positive, maintains enthusiasm	Positive, but hesitant; requires some feedback	No response to feedback	Negative, disheartened; requires much feedback	Very negative, rejects feedback
Attention	Attentive and focused	Focused, but distractible at times	Distractible, but can be refocused, needs prompting	Distracted, and difficult to refocus	Distracted and off task
Compliance	Cooperative	Insecure	Hesitant	Uncooperative	Refusing
Comments					

General DA report template

The template may be used in conjunction with any assessment to summarise the findings of the DA under headings specifically relevant to a DA, as described in Chapter 6.

Assessment report

Name ....   Date ....

Assessor ....   Place ....

The child was assessed using the dynamic assessment of. . .

A dynamic test is one that helps the child with prompts and cues throughout the test in order to assess the child's potential to learn from the practice of doing the test items and from the assistance of the examiner. It enables the examiner to find out not only what language structures are difficult for the child but also what he understands about the language structures and rules, how he approaches a difficult task and what kind of cues help him to succeed.

In this test, the child was required to. . .

Findings of the DA
Observations of language problem-solving skills

1 *Detail of language structures that the child has difficulty with, which is additional to that obtained from the standardised tests*

2 *The child's ability to transfer, or generalise, learning or strategies – i.e. item – to item transfer*

3 *The child's metalinguistic knowledge, ability to label, explain and manipulate linguistic concepts*

4 *The child's metacognitive ability – i.e. awareness of the processes and strategies that are used to solve the given task*

Behavioural factors

1   *Attention /activity/ emotion while engaged in the presented task*

2   *Motivation/attitude to learning/interest/response to input, while engaged in the presented task*

3   *Use of strategies, including reliance on others for help*

Summary of learning needs

Recommendations

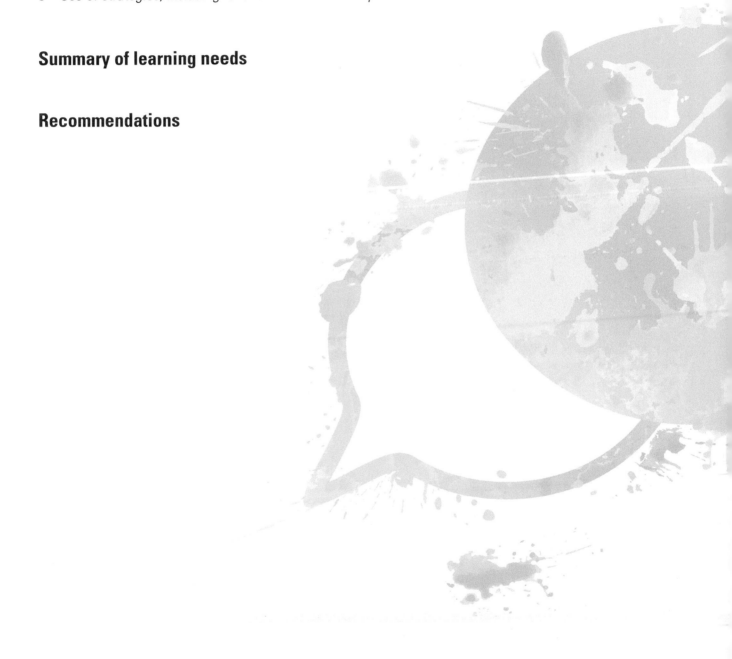

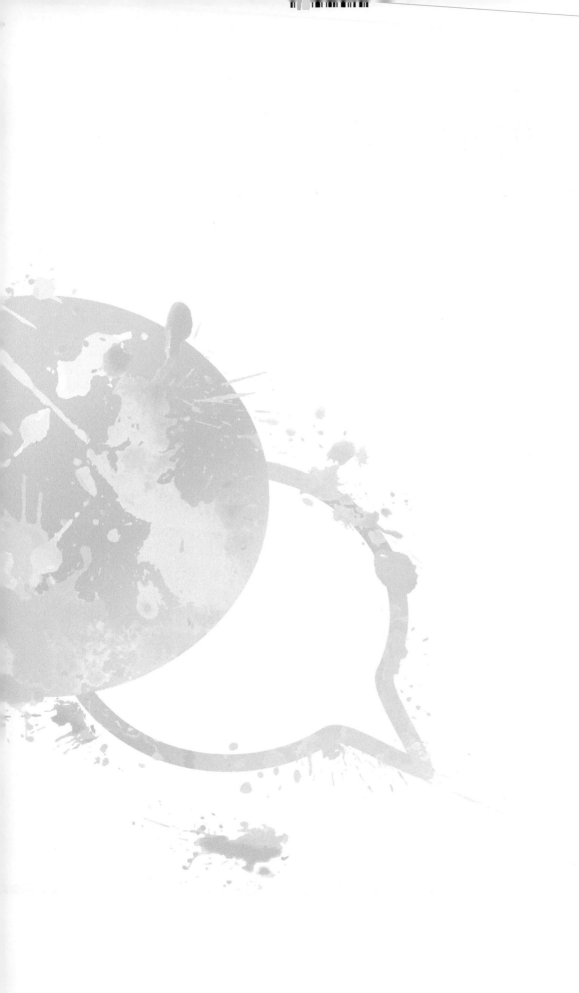

Appendix C

References for further applications of DA

References for applications of DA to other clinical populations. Other articles by the given authors are also recommended for further reading.

Alony, S., and Kozulin, A. (2007) 'Dynamic assessment of receptive language in children with Down syndrome'. *International Journal of Speech-Language Pathology*, 9(4), pp. 323–331.

Donaldson, A.L., and Olswang, L.B. (2007) 'Investigating requests for information in children with autism spectrum disorders: Static versus dynamic assessment', *International Journal of* Speech-Language *Pathology*, 9(4), pp. 297–311.

Feuerstein, R., Feuerstein, R.S., Falik, L.H. and Rand, Y. (2002) *The dynamic assessment of cognitive modifiability: The learning propensity assessment device: Theory, instruments and techniques*, ICELP Press, Jerusalem.

Haywood, H.C., and Miller, M.B. (2003) 'Dynamic assessment of adults with traumatic brain injuries', *Journal of Cognitive Education and Psychology*, 3(2), pp. 137–163.

Hasson, N. (2005) *The use of dynamic methods of language assessment in language impaired children*. Poster presented to IACEP conference, Durham UK.

Hasson, N., Nash, L., Cubie, B., Kessie, A. and Marshall, C. (2014) *Dynamic assessment of morphological analysis: A UK based Study*. Poster presented to RCSLT Conference, University of Leeds.

Hessels-Schlatter, C. (2002) 'A dynamic test to assess learning capacity in people with severe impairments', *American Journal on Mental Retardation*, 107(5), pp. 340–351.

Kaniel, S., and Tzuriel, D. (1992) 'Mediated learning experience approach in the assessment and treatment of borderline psychotic adolescents', Haywood, H.C., and Tzuriel, D. (eds) *Interactive assessment*, Springer-Verlag, New York.

Keane, K.J. (1987) 'Assessing deaf children', Lidz, C.S. (ed) *Dynamic assessment: An interactional approach to evaluating learning potential*, Guilford Press, New York.

Lantolf, J.P., and Poehner, M.E. (2004) 'Dynamic assessment of L2 development: Bringing the past into the future', *Journal of Applied Linguistics*, 1(1), pp. 49–72.

Lidz, C.S. (2004) 'Successful application of a dynamic assessment procedure with deaf students between the ages of four and eight years', *Educational and Child Psychology*, 21, pp. 59–73.

Lidz, C.S., and Elliott, J.G. (2006) 'Use of dynamic assessment with gifted students', *Gifted Education International*, 21(2), pp. 151–161.

Mann, W., Peña, E.D. and Morgan, G. (2014) 'Exploring the use of dynamic language assessment with deaf children, who use American sign language: Two case studies', *Journal of Communication Disorders*, 52, pp. 16–30.

Miller, L., Gillam, R.B. and Pena, E.D. (2001) *Dynamic assessment and intervention: Improving children's narrative abilities*, Pro-Ed, Austin, Texas.

Samuels, M.T., Lamb, C.H. and Oberholtzer, L. (1992) 'Dynamic assessment of adults with learning difficulties', Haywood, H.C., and Tzuriel, D. (eds) *Interactive assessment*, Springer-Verlag, New York.

Samuels, M.T., Tzuriel, D. and Malloy-Miller, T. (1989) 'Dynamic assessment of children with learning difficulties', Brown, R.T., and Chazan, M. (eds) *Learning difficulties and emotional problems*, Detselig, Calgary, Alberta.

Wiedl, K.H., Schöttke, H. and Garcia, M. (2001) 'Dynamic assessment of cognitive rehabilitation potential in schizophrenic persons and in elderly persons with and without dementia', *European Journal of Psychological Assessment*, 17(2), pp. 112–119.